SURVIVING DEMENTIA CARE

The Realities of Caregiving

Surviving Dementia Care is a compassionate and insightful guide for anyone navigating the challenging journey of caring for a loved one with dementia. Drawing on research from information studies, literary studies, and interviews with family caregivers, this book reimagines dementia care – not as a set of skills to master, but as a deeply human experience to endure and understand.

To make sense of the copious information on dementia, the book introduces four distinct modes of understanding dementia care, each offering a unique perspective and source of strength. The Describing mode helps caregivers grasp the medical realities of dementia. The Understanding mode addresses the shifting landscape of communication as cognitive abilities change. The Advocating mode guides readers through the complexities and anxieties of securing proper care within an often-confusing health care system. Finally, the Imagining mode reveals how creativity can foster moments of joy and connection, even in the midst of loss.

By filtering the vast array of information on dementia through these practical and empathetic modes, *Surviving Dementia Care* empowers caregivers to find the guidance they need at each stage of the journey, avoid information overload, and preserve the loving bonds that inspired their caregiving in the first place.

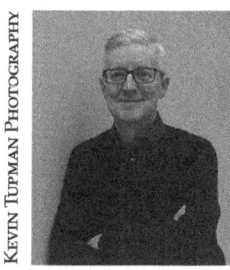

D. GRANT CAMPBELL is a professor emeritus at Western University in Canada. He taught at Queen's University, University of Toronto, and Dalhousie University, before spending 28 years on the Faculty of Information and Media Studies at Western University, where he earned two awards for excellence in teaching.

Surviving Dementia Care

The Realities of Caregiving

D. GRANT CAMPBELL

UNIVERSITY OF TORONTO PRESS
Toronto Buffalo London

University of Toronto Press
Toronto Buffalo London
utppublishing.com

© University of Toronto Press 2026

ISBN 978-1-4875-6192-5 (paper)   ISBN 978-1-4875-6194-9 (EPUB)
　　　　　　　　　　　　　　　　ISBN 978-1-4875-6193-2 (PDF)

All rights reserved. No part of this publication may be reproduced, stored in or introduced into a retrieval system, or transmitted in any form or by any means (electronic, mechanical, photocopying, recording, or otherwise) without the prior written permission of both the copyright owner and the above publisher of this book.

Library and Archives Canada Cataloguing in Publication

Title: Surviving dementia care : the realities of caregiving / D. Grant Campbell.
Names: Campbell, D. Grant, author.
Description: Includes bibliographical references and index.
Identifiers: Canadiana (print) 20250317672 | Canadiana (ebook) 20250317907 | ISBN 9781487561925 (softcover) | ISBN 9781487561949 (EPUB) | ISBN 9781487561932 (PDF)
Subjects: LCSH: Caregivers. | LCSH: Dementia – Patients – Care. | LCSH: Dementia – Patients – Home care. | LCSH: Caregivers – Psychology. | LCSH: Caregivers – Biography.
Classification: LCC RC521 .C36 2026 | DDC 362.1968/31 – dc23

Printed in Canada

Cover design: Georgie Proctor
Cover image: Shutterstock.com/Anna Hoychuk

The manufacturer's authorised representative in the EU for product safety is Mare Nostrum Group B.V., Mauritskade 21D, 1091 GC Amsterdam, The Netherlands. Email: gpsr@mare-nostrum.co.uk

We wish to acknowledge the land on which the University of Toronto Press operates. This land is the traditional territory of the Wendat, the Anishnaabeg, the Haudenosaunee, the Métis, and the Mississaugas of the Credit First Nation.

University of Toronto Press acknowledges the financial support of the Government of Canada, the Canada Council for the Arts, and the Ontario Arts Council, an agency of the Government of Ontario, for its publishing activities.

 Canada Council for the Arts / Conseil des Arts du Canada

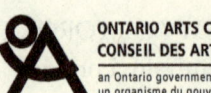 ONTARIO ARTS COUNCIL / CONSEIL DES ARTS DE L'ONTARIO
an Ontario government agency
un organisme du gouvernement de l'Ontario

Funded by the Government of Canada / Financé par le gouvernement du Canada

 MIX Paper | Supporting responsible forestry FSC® C103567

To my parents, Donald and Maida Campbell, who kept teaching us right up to the end.

And to my sisters, Allison, Leslie, Lorna, and Pegi. We worked through it together.

Contents

Preface: Turning Over the Placemat   ix
A Note on the Participants   xv
Acknowledgments   xvii

Part One – Introduction

1 Introducing Dementia Care   5
2 Introducing Modes   19

Part Two – Getting the Facts: The Describing Mode

3 Labelling Dementia   35
4 Classifying Dementia   48

Part Three – Following the Thread: The Understanding Mode

5 Conversation   65
6 Categories   80

Part Four – Taking a Stand: The Advocating Mode

7 Facing Out   95

8 Looking In   112

Part Five – Taking a Breath: The Imagining Mode

9 Creative Surges   129

10 Pleasure   142

Part Six – Closing the Distance

11 A Skeptical Pause   159

12 An Optimistic Conclusion   167

Epilogue: Learning from an Organist   181

Appendix 1: Researching Dementia as a Family Caregiver   187

Appendix 2: More about Modes   195

Notes   205

Index   217

Preface: Turning Over the Placemat

This is a book about preserving family relationships in the face of dementia. It's not a "how to" book, but it alludes to the growing body of research in dementia in various disciplines, together with the experiences of family caregivers, both in interviews and in published memoirs, and combines them in an effort to cast the family caregiving experience into some coherent shape.

When my sisters and I were growing up, my parents used to take each of us, on our birthdays, to dinner at their favorite restaurant. It was an opportunity, rare in a large family, for my parents to spend time with one of their children apart from the other four. As I moved into my teenage years and started planning my future life, these dinners were scenes of important discussions. What lay after high school? What kind of life would I make for myself as I became an adult? What choices would I make in the years ahead?

Inevitably, my father would turn over his paper placemat, haul out a pen, and start plotting out my life in rows and columns, laying out my future like a game of Solitaire. As we ate our dinner, he methodically enumerated the skill sets to cultivate for various careers, the factors to consider in the choice of a school, the things to look for when hunting for an apartment in a new city. By the time we reached dessert, he had drawn a diagram of my life, classified and enumerated in systematic order, and for a while at least, everything linked together and everything made sense.

As I grew up, I learned to do this on my own, and as a librarian who teaches librarians, I have come to admire those who drag order out of chaos. After all, it was a nineteenth-century librarian named Melvil Dewey who divided all of human knowledge into ten classes, each divided into ten divisions, and each division into ten sections. The results look much like the back of my father's placemat, and libraries across the globe use the Dewey Decimal System to this day. And in the 1990s, a scientist at CERN named Tim Berners-Lee sketched out a rough concept map of a proposed system of organizing the internet, one that resulted in the World Wide Web. You can do amazing things if you like sorting things into categories, even if you have only a placemat or the back of an envelope on which to draw your diagrams.

When both my parents developed dementia, my sisters and I had to turn over the placemat once again and organize our parents' predicament as best we could. The book that follows this preface was written in the same spirit as those diagrams that organized my life over dinner all those years ago. By combining the findings of various bodies of research and weaving in the experience of family caregivers, this book attempts to impose some order upon a phenomenon that appears to defy order, one that has invaded many, many lives.

As I tell my students every year, if you're going to organize information, you have to define three things: what you're organizing, why you're going to the trouble of doing so, and how you're dividing it up. In this case, I'm not seeking to impose order on dementia *per se*, but on the experience of caring for someone who is living with dementia. Furthermore, I am primarily concerned not with institutional caregiving in long-term care facilities, but with the lay caregiving provided by family members for someone that they love. And the reason for doing this is to help families preserve that love as long as possible. Dementia brings about devastating changes in family life; if this book can help family members sustain a loving relationship in the face of such changes, it will have served its purpose.

As for how I'm dividing things up, the organizational plan of this book rests on some basic observations. First, I take it as a given that dementia is an inherently bad piece of luck. It is not a blessing in disguise; for all the silver linings we may find, dementia remains an unpleasant, exhausting, and deeply sad experience both for the person living with it and the people who provide the support and care. For that reason, family caregivers need as much help as we can give them.

Second, dementia is a fiendishly complicated phenomenon that has generated active research in various disciplines. There's no shortage of information about dementia. Scholarly journals in medicine and psychology and nursing abound with findings from a multitude of studies. Personal memoirs both by people with dementia and by their caregivers offer their personal stories. Alzheimer societies across the globe offer advice and services and opportunities for information sharing both in person and online. If you're one of those people who like drinking from a firehose, dementia care will be right up your alley.

Unfortunately, most of us don't much like drinking from a firehose. What's more, dementia care isn't a skill we master, so much as an experience we survive, and we have to be ruthless in distinguishing information that meets the needs of the moment from that which doesn't. Because dementia complicates life in so many different ways, a caregiver must approach dementia from different directions, depending on the need of the moment. And we need to organize the information available to us according to the direction of approach: not to pose as experts, but to emerge as survivors.

To that end, I offer four primary directions from which to approach the various tasks of dementia care, which I term "modes." The first mode I call the **"describing mode"**: establishing the truth of the situation according to what we call "the real world." This is the world, not just of scientific and medical fact, but of the facts of the social world around us. This approach predominates particularly at the time of diagnosing the illness, in which the loved one's various symptoms – forgetfulness, mood changes, trouble with words – are explained according to scientific and medical knowledge, procedure and definitions, together with all the legal, social, and economic consequences that follow. The second mode, **"understanding,"** tries to understand our loved ones on their own terms, rather than measuring them against the world of external facts. We take this tack when we converse with loved ones who break many rules of normal conversation, whose statements are not strictly true, whose language has become distorted, or whose actions seem to defy logic or common sense. With the third mode, **"advocating,"** we confront the necessity of advocating on behalf of our loved ones to medical and health care systems. This becomes particularly important when deciding when and where to place our loved ones in long-term care. At such times, we are surrounded by repeated professions of care and concern, and our skepticism about these professions leads us to examine our own commitments to the loved one's best interests.

Each of these approaches becomes useful at various times in the caregiving process. Each as well contains a crucial ambiguity at its heart: moments when its internal logic appears to break down and leave us more perplexed than ever. The fourth and final mode, **"imagining,"** occurs through activities that are repeated frequently, to the point where they become a form of ritual. Such activities can be as simple as brushing the loved one's hair, dancing to music on the radio, making a pot of tea, taking a walk, or singing a song. In this approach, both caregiver and loved one participate in a shared activity that absorbs the complexities of the three former approaches but somehow makes them tolerable. While I deal primarily with the example of music in this book, music is by no means the only activity in which this phenomenon occurs. This approach tends to be occasional and sporadic, but in some ways the most meaningful.

Let me close this preface with a few disclaimers. First, the approaches I define emerged from my own background in both librarianship and literary studies. As such, they have a special meaning for me, and they manage, at least on some level, to make sense of the confusion we encounter in dementia care. But I've worked in libraries long enough to realize that some of the best moments in a library occur not when people learn the system but when they learn to resist it. If the limitations of my categories inspire you to form ones that work better for you, the book will have done its work.

Second, while the focus is on dementia caregiving, this will not be a guide to specific methods of caregiving, nor a directory of support systems or institutional resources. Health care systems vary from country to country, as well as within countries, and are subject to rapid changes over time. Because I am Canadian, the book will inevitably reflect the Canadian health care context: all of my interview participants are Canadian, as are the authors of the memoirs I cite. But the caregiving experience, as I am addressing it, applies very widely. This book will hopefully enable a caregiver to recognize which resources – be they library programs, Alzheimer societies, doctors, social workers, or support groups – are appropriate for the specific approach that is needed to address a particular challenge.

Finally, while I hope this book helps caregivers retain loving relationships with their family members for as long as possible, I'm fully aware that this is sometimes impossible. Dementia is a ravaging disease that can render a person totally helpless, and in some cases wreak drastic changes in the loved one's personality and typical responses. If your loved one has changed to the point where it is no longer possible to retain the intimacy and closeness of former times, do not let any part of this book prevent you from taking sensible measures to protect your health and well-being, and that of your family.

If, on the other hand, you believe that the story of your relationship is not yet over, perhaps this book will help. My sisters and I were fortunate, indeed: we continued learning from our parents right up to the end, and while I wouldn't wish the task of dementia care on anyone, nor do I regret my own experience of it. I merely wish to turn over the placemat and sketch it out, in hopes that others might benefit from what I've learned.

A Note on the Participants

Ten people appear in this study, identified simply by pseudonyms: George, Ben, Fred, Lydia, Tina, Jeff, Victor, Mary, Jane, and Nancy. While our interviews adhered to, and were approved by, the ethics rules at Western University, I'd be misleading you if I suggested that these were full-on qualitative interviews of the type one sees in the social sciences. My conversations with these people were open-ended conversations with a bare minimum of structure, and my data analysis consisted of listening to their voices, watching their faces and revisiting the transcripts as I absorbed their accounts as well as I could.

The men and women I spoke to were all, or had recently been, caregivers to someone close to them. George, Ben, and Fred had until recently been caring for a mother, while Lydia and Patricia were still caring for theirs. Mary had recently lost her father, while Victor was still caring for his; Jeff was caring for his husband, and Nancy was caring for a loved friend in her religious community. Jane had recently lost two parents to dementia and was now dealing with her husband's failing cognition.

Our conversations were deep and rich; as many qualitative researchers will tell you, the generosity with which people share their experiences is deeply moving. The interviews yielded many insights that appear in the book as particular instances or experiences. But the interviews pervade the book in a less obvious way, through the various emotional states that the participants revealed: stoic acceptance, deep anger, retrospective fondness, retrospective weariness, laughter tinged with tears, tears tinged with laughter. Observing these emotional responses, together with those expressed in the published memoirs, enabled me to establish a bridge between my own personal experiences on the one hand and the empirical research on the other. I am deeply grateful to them.

Acknowledgments

This research was made possible through funding from the Rogers Chair of Studies in Journalism and New Information Technology, which I held from 2013 to 2015, and from an Insight Development Grant from the Social Sciences and Humanities Research Council of Canada. I completed it within the supportive and stimulating intellectual environment of the Faculty of Information and Media Studies at Western University in London, Ontario.

Various communities deserve my warmest thanks. I'm indebted to the various chapters of the International Society for Knowledge Organization, and particularly to the ISKO-Brazil chapter, as well as to the Federal University of Paraná in Brazil, for providing the opportunity to air my research at various stages. The Information Architecture community also provided supportive opportunities for me to explore my research in its early stages. In addition to these academic communities, I'm also indebted to Metropolitan United Church in Toronto, to the Inter-Generational Choir, formed through the Alzheimer's Association of London-Middlesex, and to the supportive care workers and staff at the King Gardens Retirement Home in Mississauga, and the Chelsey Park Extended Care Facility in Streetsville.

As for individuals, it's difficult to know where to begin, let alone where to stop. In the journalism faculty at Western, Meredith Levine provided me with my first opportunity to explore issues of dementia, and shared the Rogers Chair with me for two years. I'm deeply grateful to her and to the student colleagues who worked with me at various times: Dr. Nicole Dalmer, Ariel Vanderschans, Dr. Sarah Cornwell, Jason Andrews, and Rebecca Power.

Throughout the length of the project, some colleagues joined the ranks of friends and witnesses as they listened patiently while I worked through the various problems. Dr. Karl Fast, Dr. José-Augusto Guimarães, and Dr. Andre Vieira Freitas de Araujo all gave generously of their time and advice. Dr. Alex Mayhew has stimulated my thinking in many ways through his unconventional views regarding the ethics of conventional discourse on aging. My closest friend at Western, Dr. Jacquelyn Burkell, has had my back from the very beginning and given unstintingly from her generous reserves of enthusiasm, curiosity, and practical advice.

On the home front, various friends have served as witnesses, not just to my experiences of dementia care but to my experiences of writing the book, including Nair Hassan, Rosa Bergman, Helen Jacob-Stein, the late Bob Benson, and the whole Benson gang: Ian, Larry, Janette, and their families.

My own family has been cheering me on throughout: not just the sisters I list in the dedication, but their husbands and their children. Particular thanks to Michelle Hundt, who read and commented on an early draft of this book, and to Dr. Harry O'Halloran for his insights not just into dementia but into health care in general. Most of all, I thank my husband, the Rev. Daniel Benson. Without him, my parents' dementia would still have happened. With his loving, patient, and supportive presence, I was able to make a few good things happen as well.

SURVIVING DEMENTIA CARE

PART ONE

Introduction

Things fall apart; the centre cannot hold;
　　　　　– William Butler Yeats[1]

For me the distressing part of dementia is what it does to the family unit.
　　　　　　　　　　　　　　　　　　– Participant Fred

CHAPTER ONE

Introducing Dementia Care

*Absent thee from felicity awhile
And in this harsh world draw thy breath in pain
To tell my story.*
— Hamlet, 5.2.331–3

This book is about personal dementia care: bearing painful witness to the story of a family member or close friend who is facing the permanent and irretrievable loss of cognitive faculties. More specifically, this book is about making sense of this experience by lending coherence to a caregiving process that often appears to lack any coherence whatsoever: a process in which, as Mike Barnes describes it, "every decision is on the fly and inexact and behind the moment."[1] By applying principles of knowledge organization to both dementia research and firsthand accounts, I classify the caregiving experience around four primary approaches, which I call "modes." Understanding these modes will not change the terminal outcome of dementia; nor are they likely to alleviate the day-to-day stress of caregiving. But if I am successful, enumerating these four modes will assist both carer and care recipient in shielding their loving relationship from dementia's corrosive effects. In addition, I hope that these modes will assist libraries, community centers, and other helping organizations to design programs of value for alleviating caregiver stress.

Families to the Rescue

We've all seen the statistics and the metaphors that accompany them. We're facing a "tsunami" of dementia around the world, a "tidal wave" of suffering as the world's population ages, a burgeoning crisis that threatens to overwhelm our economies and our societies. According to the World Health Organization, by 2021, 55 million people worldwide were living with dementia, with that number expected to rise to 78 million in 2030 and 139 million by 2050.[2]

We've all witnessed what is happening to our infrastructures of health care. Even before army units were drafted into nursing homes to perform basic care during the COVID pandemic, we watched besieged nursing home administrators explaining how persistent staff shortages were making it next to impossible to cover shifts adequately. Budget shortfalls, widespread retirements in the nursing and medical professions, wait times, poor access to physicians: the nightly news gives us unrelenting pictures of a health system riddled with neglect, shortage, and inadequacy.

With dementia on the rise, and with health care systems stretched to capacity, family members will be called in to fill the gap. Indeed, there is no question in anyone's mind: if you are caring for a family member with dementia, you are not a bystander or an ornament to our current predicament. You are a fundamental player. If Canada and other countries survive this demographic wave of suffering, much of the credit will go to people like you.

For that reason, support for family caregivers figures prominently in Canada's National Dementia Strategy:

> Often, family members, neighbours and friends care for someone living with dementia, and organize the care delivered by others. These caregivers help with the essential activities of daily living and help keep the person living with dementia engaged in activities ... Caregivers are essential members of the care team; improving support for them is integral to improving the quality of life of the person they are caring for and to ensuring their own health.[3]

The present book aligns with this particular arm of Canada's strategy for dealing with dementia, one that appears in numerous provincial strategies as well. It aims to provide support for "essential members of the care team": support directed at those who are caring for a family member – a parent, a spouse, a friend – out of love, obligation, and shared history.

The caring can arise from different causes; there are many kinds of dementia, with many different symptoms, which appear in different combinations and intensities with each individual. The caring can also arise in different locations: the loved one might be living in the same home as the carer, or live alone or with someone else, or be in some form of assisted living. The caring probably involves a multitude of different tasks, at least some of which the caregiver feels less than competent to carry out. But despite this intimidating variety, this book is written for those with a common motivation: caregiving that arises not from a vocational choice but from a long-term, loving relationship.

And the book's theme is survival: not of the caregiver, specifically, but of that deep commitment that made the person a caregiver in the first place.

The Need for Information

The chapters that follow spring from an insight that is painfully obvious to just about everyone: caring for someone with dementia is a difficult and unpleasant experience. Yes, there are bright moments, meaningful moments, profound moments, and yes, we can look back with some nostalgia on the experience afterwards, just as we can upon many bad experiences that we survived to remember. But every happy moment emerges against a backdrop of difficult, depressing, anxiety-provoking, exasperating labor, as the caregiver wearily adapts to change after change after change in the loved one's situation. Many caregivers, I hope, look back on their work with pride. But few, I suspect, looked forward to the prospect at the outset. And few indeed, I am sure, emerged without scars of some kind.

To support caregivers through this painful experience, Canada's dementia strategy identifies information as a key resource:

- Supporting the mental and physical health and wellbeing of caregivers by identifying, and sharing evidence-informed, culturally safe and culturally appropriate information, tools and resources on, for example: self-care; how to navigate the health care system; approaching primary care practitioners about symptoms or concerns; how to provide care for a person living with dementia; and how to support transitions to long-term care.

- Continuing to fund community-based projects on mental health supports and information about self-care for caregivers as well as promoting the use of available respite services and community support groups.[4]

Clearly, the strategy states, our national cohort of family caregivers constitutes an essential resource that needs protection. We need to provide access to relief from the strain, by providing home care options, as well as chances for the caregiver to get away from time to time to decompress. We also need to provide appropriate treatments and therapies to address the caregiver's scars, in the form of depression, substance abuse and other psychological and medical consequences. First and foremost, we need to facilitate access to information about dementia, about caregiving, and about the resources available.

Few would quarrel with the need for information. There is much to learn when caring for a loved one with dementia: the condition pulls the caregiver into areas of medical research regarding the symptoms, causes, and treatment of different kinds of dementia; legal regulations around asset management and powers of attorney; regulations and procedures for obtaining home care. The caregiver often needs to become a lay expert in physiotherapy, geriatrics, home maintenance, computer technology, pharmacy, and fraud prevention. And this doesn't include all the other little things one learns: how to navigate the various payment systems in different hospital parking lots, which elevator to take, and how to fit a wheelchair into the back of a car.

If the problems of dementia caregiving are overwhelming, the information available for solving them can be daunting as well. For one thing, there's lots of it. Dementia was once a delicate secret in many families, hiding behind euphemisms like "scatty" and "dotty." Recent years have witnessed a proliferation of discourse surrounding dementia: guides, informational websites, social media support groups, peer-reviewed articles, data archives, research institutes, infomercials, bureaucratic procedures at all levels of government, societies, and conferences. We may be a long way from finding a cure for dementia, but we certainly know how to write about it and talk about it.

For the caregiver, much of this information can be embarrassing, depressing, and downright frightening. Questions around geriatric sexuality aren't everyone's chosen topic of discussion; nor are concerns of privacy, driving safety, money management, living wills, aphasia, sundowning, personality change, or incontinence. We may be grateful to have access to government regulations regarding geriatric drivers' tests, but it's no fun contemplating that day when the loved one must surrender up the car keys. And while Western culture has become far more open about discussing intimate bodily functions, not all of us are ready to drop our reticence, especially when the discussion concerns parents or spouses.

As if that weren't enough, much of the most pressing information comes at awkward moments: often in real-time exchanges, either face-to-face or online, that require interpretation and responses without the leisure to read and absorb. We have consultations with doctors after the loved one has had a fall; with social workers and geriatricians while the spouse is restless to return home; with administrators, accountants, and lawyers while we're trying to deal with home care that has fallen through. Many of us must confer with other family members, who are sometimes at different stages of realization and acceptance of the problem, or located far away and therefore need us to relay information to them. Above all, we have interactions with the loved one, interactions that grow increasingly baffling as the dementia progresses, causing deep shifts in memory patterns, moods, and sometimes personality.

Research into information use tells us that there's nothing especially new about information overload, nor are caregivers the only group that feels daunted by the task of learning how to find and use information. Most of us, at some time in our lives, have experienced that state of vertigo, where a seemingly simple task blossoms into helpless confusion, the moment we start to look things up. Problems can look clear from a distance, but once we start investigating them up close, the things we learn make us less sure of ourselves. We discover conflicting opinions and contradictory perspectives; every new piece of information we acquire puzzles us more, and that crystalline decision we were hoping for seems to get further and further away, separated by bewilderment and doubt. Researchers have traced this process in various cases of information-seeking. And reference librarians frequently witness the frustration of people who seek a simple answer, only to discover that there's no simple answer available.

The vertigo of the caregiver, however, is special in some ways. First, dementia care isn't something you solve once; things may stay stable for a time, but inevitably the loved one's condition changes, necessitating a whole new round of learning. As Mike Barnes puts it in his memoir of caregiving, the changes are rarely neatly defined: "[the stages] are taking place in a person, with all her quirks and qualities; … she is as subject to the vicissitudes of mood and physical health and events of the day and even weather as the rest of us."[5] Second, the challenges of dementia care go on for a long time; it's like writing a high school essay that takes ten years to complete. Here's Mike Barnes again: "Not a crisis, but a life. How does a crisis become a life?"[6]

And finally, the inevitable conclusion is hardly an attractive one, such as a finished essay or a new house or a fresh skill that opens opportunities. Dementia care ends when the loved one dies, leaving us with grief, together with a lot of accumulated experience doing things we weren't trained to do, and which few of us are eager to cultivate in a new setting.

What, then, do caregivers need in order to master this sad and bewildering situation? To be sure, they need information, but they also need some support in using it. What does that support look like?

The Need for a Sense of Competence

Two influential psychologists in self-determination theory, Richard Ryan and Edward Deci, argue that all of us have basic psychological needs which must be fed from "specific nutrients in the social environment" if we are to lead healthy lives. In particular, all of us need an environment that enables us to evolve a sense of competence: "our basic need to feel effectance and mastery. People need to feel able to operate effectively within their important life contexts."[7] It's not so much about knowing things as knowing how to get along in life with a sense that you're doing things well. And let's face it: most family caregivers are not formally trained in many of the tasks that confront them. There's a reason why doctors go to medical school, not to mention all the training undergone by nurses and therapists and lawyers and nutritionists and physiotherapists and gerontologists. They spent money and time learning how to do jobs that you're doing on the fly. It's difficult to keep a loved one safe and happy and healthy when physical tasks that ordinarily call for a trained expert leave you exhausted, or when you're daunted by a constant fear that you could be doing something wrong. And the helplessness we feel at the bewildering array of tasks that face us can be a major source of debilitating depression and anxiety.

Psychologists have determined that categories and schemas help to alleviate this sense of demoralizing ineptitude. Schemas are mental models that we store in our heads that help us remember things and cope with the world.[8] We learn to recognize recurring patterns in life, which enable us to establish workable categories of things that share some common characteristics. We may be facing an unfamiliar task, but that task may be similar in some ways to other tasks we've mastered in the past. Arraying these categories in a working order enables us to achieve "cognitive economy," in which we can usefully transfer our acquired knowledge of one situation to another.[9] Like the back-of-the-envelope diagrams we draw during a brainstorming meeting, or the diagrams and lists laid out on a turned-over placemat during a working lunch, some kind of working schema of the caregiving process gives the caregiver a sense of order, out of which a sense of competence can gradually evolve. I call that sense of order "coherence."

The Need for Coherence

In a world where we celebrate quests for money, for conquest, for a lover, or for a Holy Grail, the quest for coherence doesn't sound too glamorous. Nonetheless, many of us sag from time to time under a pervasive sense that the world and its workings are unfathomable. In my years of studying English literature, I used to bump up frequently against the word "muddle." Characters like Stephen Blackpool in Dickens's *Hard Times* or Lucy Honeychurch in Forster's *A Room with a View* find themselves in "a muddle": a state of helpless confusion in the face of multiple worries and conflicting demands that threaten to overwhelm them. And in the musical *A Little Night Music*, the world-weary

Desirée Armfeldt looks over her life and longs "to turn back, to find some sort of coherent existence after so many years of muddle."[10]

Coherence was described by Samuel Johnson in 1755 as that state in which one part of a discourse neither destroys nor contradicts another.[11] It's an attractive concept, and one very helpful for getting through the day. Life falls into patterns of regularity, and those patterns give us some power to predict what's going to happen next. Buses and trains arrive at their prescribed stations; people show up for work; stores open in the morning and close at night. On some basic level, the chunks of life fit together without contradiction, and the world makes sense.

It doesn't pay to look too closely at these patterns on which we rely. Coherence can be false; it can be limited. When the sun gives every appearance of coming up in the day and going down at night, it's awfully easy to assume that the sun is circling the Earth, rather than the other way around. Nonetheless, within its limits, we can predict, along with George Carlin's Hippy-Dippy Weatherman, that the weather at night will be "dark, turning partly light by morning."[12] Family dynamics within a household acquire a similar regularity: the people who share our lives over a long period often prove to have regular times of rising in the morning, recurring appetites for certain foods, familiar tastes in music, and predictable patterns of conversation.

Cases of dementia often begin to manifest themselves as tiny disruptions in these states of mundane coherence: oddities of behavior or utterance that increasingly undermine our ability to predict the loved one's behavior. The consequences can touch all aspects of the person's life: behavior at work, management of finances, ability to shop or cook, or participation in leisure activities. The caregiver's life too becomes increasingly unpredictable, as a formerly settled routine is punctured by calls from the police to collect someone who got lost on the way home, kitchen fires from neglected cooking, and sudden mood swings. As the caregiver's ability to understand and predict the most basic events of daily life erodes steadily, the suggested diagnoses and solutions come from many different directions. Explanations can vary and be completely wrong; a declining interest in social interaction can be diagnosed as depression, and a failure to recognize familiar landmarks as poor eyesight. As the loved one's dementia progresses, so do the complexities, the speculations, the uncertainties, the unexpected challenges, and the moments of exhaustion. Throughout it all, the caregiver is tempted to sigh, along with Dickens's Stephen Blackpool, "It's all a muddle."

There Is Help Out There

But there is help, and this book attempts to put some of that help into coherent order by drawing on sources of assistance that caregivers themselves may be too busy or too exhausted to find for themselves.

We are witnessing a growing number of memoirs written by caregivers, and this book makes extensive use of three of them: *Enter Mourning* by Heather Menzies (2009), *The Long Hello* by Cathie Borrie (2015), and *Be With* by Mike Barnes (2018). I chose these particular memoirs for a number of reasons. First, like me, they are Canadian and reflect a Canadian health care context that I can recognize. Second, all three of them use the experience of dementia care as a gateway into broader speculations: on the nature of family, of love, of loyalty, of responsibility. These speculations haunt family caregivers constantly, and these memoirs give voice to them. Finally, each provides a separate and distinct approach. Menzies, a journalist, delves into the science that underlies the descriptive mode. Borrie's exploration of the patterns and music of her mother's spoken words give us an entry into the understanding mode, while Barnes brings a poet's lyricism to questions of loyalty and solidarity that underlie the advocating mode. Like many such memoirs, these accounts give eloquent testimony of a caregiver's urgent need to put the entire bewildering experience into some kind of coherent structure. All too often, such perspective is gained only after the loved one has passed away, leaving the caregiver with the mental and emotional room to process the experience. I hope, in this book, to honor the generosity of these three authors, and to help make their insights useful and sustaining to those who are struggling through what they have survived.

This book also draws on ten conversations I held with present and former caregivers within my own community. Some were in the thick of caregiving; others were reflecting on the experience after the loved one's death. Some were spouses; some were children; one was a member of a religious community, caring for a fellow member. They spoke frankly of their experiences, both good and bad; they spoke lovingly of the person in their care; they spoke honestly about their encounters with systems of health care and elder care. Their testimonies speak to the range of problems faced by family caregivers, and to the patterns of similarity that emerge among them.

Finally, this book draws on research. Dementia research has become an industry in nearly every faculty across the modern university, and this can be a problem. Universities and research centers are producing far more scholarly output than any caregiver could hope to absorb. Many of these studies use specific and rigorous research methods, employing specialist language and drawing on complex theories and a long series of previous studies. Many studies produce highly tentative results, surrounded by the caution and refusal to infer widely that characterizes empirical research in a complex phenomenon. Above all, much of it necessarily strives to understand the effects of dementia on the persons living with the condition, rather than on their caregivers. Nonetheless, I believe that this research can help caregivers, if mobilized and presented in the right way. In this book, I am drawing on my own expertise – in literary studies, librarianship, and knowledge organization – in an attempt to map out a potential "right way."

In librarianship, we often make a distinction between general and special information centers. A general information center is something like a public library: you get information on everything under the sun, and people use it for all kinds of reasons. In a special library, by contrast, you collect information in a specific area, and people use it for specific and defined purposes.[13] Dementia care within families is a general problem masquerading as a specialized one. It looks like a limited set of needs, needing a limited set of information. But scratch the surface, and you find that caregivers need information on a bewildering range of topics, and they need them at highly varying times. What's more, as caregivers become more experienced, they develop a formidable lay expertise, becoming experts in areas where they previously felt helpless, skeptical about things they formerly believed, and suspicious of information sources that they formerly trusted implicitly. And like most of us when we've been stretched beyond our limits, they don't always have a lot of patience.

Nonetheless, I'm writing this book because I believe it is possible, with some care and some artful organization, to set at least some of the voluminous research on dementia alongside the written and oral testimonies of caregivers. In the chapters that follow, I will lay out a method for categorizing, organizing, and surviving the personal caregiving experience. I hope it will open up other possibilities for strengthening the endurance of both caregiver and care recipient, and for preserving what most deserves protection: a longstanding bond of love and respect.

CHAPTER TWO

Introducing Modes

Chess. When one is outmatched, the game is over. Checkmate.
...
Not chess, Mr. Spock. Poker.

– *Star Trek*[1]

When I was an undergraduate student at University of Toronto, I took a course on Shakespeare with Northrop Frye. Frye was a respected, even revered scholar, and the class was huge; apart from a few timid questions in the lecture hall, I never spoke to him directly. But I enjoyed his lectures. He spoke gently and with dry humor; his deadpan plot summary of that Shakespearean bloodbath, *Titus Andronicus*, had us all in hysterics. Only a few years later, he became a national celebrity, when *The Great Code*, the first of his two books on the Bible and literature, hit the bestseller lists, alongside *The Jane Fonda Workout Book*.

If Northrop Frye were alive today, he'd be astounded, and perhaps offended, to catch me making use of his theories in a book on dementia. If so, I apologize to his shade, but I'm a librarian who specializes in knowledge organization, and Northrop Frye is a librarian's dream. He moves into massive, complex, tangled areas of knowledge and puts them in order. Whether it's the poetry of William Blake, the drama of Shakespeare, Canadian literature, world literature, or the Bible, Frye goes in and sets to work. He establishes categories. He extracts patterns. In his own words, he works to reveal an underlying coherence to areas of human thought that appear tangled, wild, and impenetrable. And after reading his work, I would turn to my copy of Blake's poetry, or my two massive volumes of the *Norton Anthology of English Literature*, and think to myself, "I can do this. This is starting to make sense." If you put this book down with a similar feeling, I'll be very proud indeed.

Nonetheless, addressing dementia care from the perspective of literature and the arts may seem unusual, in light of all the information that comes out of medicine and psychology and nursing. When a caregiver is too tired to read the newspaper in the morning, what use is literature?

Why the Arts? And Why Imaginative Literature?

"In the middle of the journey of our life, I came to myself within a dark wood where the straight way was lost."

– Dante[2]

If someone you love – if someone on whom you've always depended – has just received a diagnosis of dementia, you might well relate to that sentence: that sense of finding yourself lost in a dark, perplexing, and terrifying landscape, with no idea what to do next.

Dante wrote that sentence back in the fourteenth century, and the rest of his three-volume *Divine Comedy* slowly releases the narrator from the fear and confusion of that forest by taking him through a sequence of structured landscapes: Hell, Purgatory, and Heavenly Paradise. In each of these landscapes, he has a guide – Virgil for the first two, and then Beatrice in Paradise – who walks with him and explains the many beautiful and terrifying things they witness. And in the centuries since, reader after reader has found consolation by following Dante along the same path.

The Divine Comedy is only one example of a durable phenomenon. Throughout the centuries, we find literary and artistic works that become friends to us as we work our way through a perplexing and frightening world. For author and journalist Rebecca Mead, George Eliot's *Middlemarch* has been a lifelong companion: a key text by which she could interpret her own life.[3] Generations of enthusiasts have immersed themselves in J.R.R. Tolkien's Middle Earth, the voyages of the starship *Enterprise*, and the heroics of the Marvel universe. And generations of readers have taken refuge in the genius of Agatha Christie's Hercule Poirot, who gathers the baffled characters together at the end of the narrative, separates the truths from the lies, discards the red herrings, and identifies the killer.

How does this help with dementia care? Beyond the sheer comfort value of snatching a moment or two with a book that's become an old friend, imaginative works often tell stories, stories that lead us into psychological places where words often fail us in real life: fantasy and frustration, unspoken fears and suppressed anxieties. They thereby enable us to get some cognitive grasp, not just of our assured principles, but also our anxieties, dreams and nightmares. Dementia is a real-life phenomenon, to be sure, but the prospect of coping with it can release nightmares: vivid mental pictures of dire possibilities. We can imagine a loved one getting lost or causing a car accident; we can visualize moments when the loved one fails to recognize us. Perhaps worst of all, we can imagine disasters that arise from our own failures of vigilance. Such visions can torment us if we don't acknowledge them and address them.

As dementia comes to occupy a more prominent place in today's cultural landscape, we are witnessing more and more narratives and memoirs and blog posts, all striving, like *Hamlet's* Horatio, to draw their breath in pain to tell the story. And there's no question that these stories matter. We need to hear the accounts of people who have traditionally been left out of the mainstream narratives that dominate our culture. That includes people who are living with dementia. It also includes the people who are caring for them. This book will feature stories: both published memoirs and narrative accounts of family caregivers.

Stories, however, have their limits. They can be a bit too tidy, a bit too easily resolved. *Law and Order* is a great show, but it does make us expect that heinous crimes can be detected, solved, tried and convicted in an hour, with commercial breaks and "thump thump" scene changes. Poirot always solves the crime; rom coms end with the lovers collapsing into each other's arms.

Dementia care is not tidy. It refuses to confine itself to a single hour in your busy schedule; it offers only vague timeframes for the different stages, and there's no way to fast-forward through the messy bits. Canadian novelist Kyo Maclear warns us not to yield to a "general cultural impatience" towards a phenomenon like dementia care that "does not unfold or dynamically change or tidily resolve": we need "to value the parts of lived experience that do not fit into a narrative shape."[4] What lies beyond stories that might enable us to value such elusive, non-narrative aspects?

As a librarian, and as a researcher in knowledge organization, I believe that we need to arrange the stories, organize them and classify them in a meaningful array. The narratives surrounding dementia can become a cacophony to the exhausted caregiver: voices upon voices upon voices, some urgent, some gentle, some erudite, some lengthy, some short, some hopeful, some relentlessly ill-tempered. Looking for helpful information on dementia sometimes feels like standing in the middle of a vast supermarket, unable to find anything to eat, or in the midst of a vast library and unable to find anything to read.

Here's where literary studies comes to the rescue once again. In all of his major work, Northrop Frye was a notorious classifier. What's more, his schemes exhibit a harmony and symmetry worthy of Dante: gently revolving miracles of balance. In Frye's work, everything has its place, and even the most confusing and dense texts, such as James Joyce's *Ulysses*, fall obediently into line. Frye makes literature, and by extension the world, look coherent. Classification, Frye argued, is an essential part of any complex discipline and any complex field of thought.

Well, caring for a loved one with dementia care is as complex as any field of study you care to name. And if Frye's methods of sorting out literature are of any help, I'm darned well going to use them. In particular, I intend to use Frye's theory of modes as a means of making sense out of the act of caring for a loved one with dementia.

What Is a Mode?

"Mode" is an old concept, with roots in grammar, philosophy and music, and if you're interested in the background, I've provided one in an appendix. As I'm using the term in this book, a mode is a way of approach. If you think of it in travelling terms, it's rather like deciding whether to take the quick highway or a scenic back road to your destination, whether to approach your destination from the main driveway that gives you the full front view or by the back way that brings you to the service entrance, whether to ring the front doorbell or to go around to the back and let yourself in with a knock and a loud "hello!" Each of these decisions involves a certain frame of mind and a certain set of assumptions and a certain background "mood."[5]

When you're caring for a loved one with dementia, you have to approach each challenge by different roads and enter by different doors. Sometimes the loved one is relatively normal, and you can play the role you've always played. At other times, you're a nurse; sometimes, unfortunately, a prison guard; sometimes a walking encyclopedia of everything the person has forgotten: husband, wife, private secretary, son, daughter, receptionist, chauffer, fashion consultant, cook – the list goes on. And each role requires you to approach it in a certain way, in a certain mood. Equally important, each role judges some information to be relevant and other information little or no help at all. If you've ever wondered why a neighbor's advice or a doctor's orders or a hospital procedure or a government regulation made perfect sense on one day and seemed irrelevant or intrusive on the next, it's probably because you were working and thinking in different modes at different times. As Captain Kirk realized on the bridge of the Starship Enterprise, sometimes you're playing chess and sometimes poker.

If that sounds daunting, it is. But here's the good news: while the situations you're facing seem endless, the modes are not endless, wheither in literature or in dementia care. In literature, we've come to recognize that various situations lend themselves to comedy and others to tragedy. Some work best in the pages of a novel, while others work best in voices on the stage. Some belong in our living rooms on TV, while others work best on an IMAX screen. And in one of his last books, *Words with Power*, Northrop Frye pushed the concept of modes beyond the limits of what we call "literature," to argue that all verbal structures – and by extension all human interactions – fall into four modes. And these are the modes I intend to use for the remainder of this book.

Mode 1: Describing

In what he calls the descriptive mode, Frye states, "we are reading to get information about something in the world outside the book."[6] The descriptive mode aims for "objective truth," and in this mode the caregiver learns the basic science of the condition and the medical procedures for diagnosis and treatment. But the mode extends beyond the empirical science of dementia and its treatment to embrace many other demanding concerns. The "real world" of this mode is not only the world of controlled experiments and scientific journals. It also includes all those unavoidable facts about our social world. The caregiver is dealing with the logistical requirements of daily living in the real world, such as sustained and regular personal hygiene, preparing and eating meals, selecting and wearing appropriate clothing, preventing accidents or exploitation, managing the household finances, and maintaining home repairs. Added to these are fresh logistical requirements of adapting to the condition: navigating the bureaucracy of the health care system, arranging legalities such as estates, living wills and power of attorney, and learning the intricacies of hospital administration and geriatric support systems. Furthermore, in this mode, the caregiver has the unenviable task of mediating between an outside world of systems, facts, and consequences on the one hand

and, on the other, someone increasingly incapable of grasping and coping with that world.

Mode 2: Understanding

Frye calls this the "conceptual" or "dialectic" mode, in which truth is established, not beyond the text but within the text, in the logical sequence of its statements and the internal arrangement of its elements. In the conceptual/dialectic mode, we search for adherence to internal laws of logic and inference; if all humans are mortal and Socrates is a human, then we can infer that Socrates is mortal. I prefer to call my adaptation of Frye's concept the "understanding mode." When a loved one's behavior fails to make sense by the outer world's standards, we try to understand the "inner logic" of the behavior.

Searching for inner consistency makes obvious sense when that consistency leads to something that's true on the outside as well. It may seem ludicrous when dealing with someone whose behavior appears irrational. Nonetheless, this actually speaks to an urgent truth in caregiving. All behavior we witness in dementia patients occurs for a reason, and sometimes the reason lies within the person's character and history and experience. A daughter may have to explain to a bewildered doctor or care provider that her father's eccentric responses actually makes perfect sense to those who know him well.

For all one's efforts to explain and align the situation with the outer world, the caregiver sooner or later must confront the world of the person experiencing the dementia. This is the mode we enter when sitting with the person: listening, conversing, watching, trying to decipher what the loved one is saying, doing, or thinking. In the understanding mode, the caregiver is attempting to communicate in a way that makes sense to the loved one, however inconsistent their interaction may be with the real world beyond those walls.

Understanding and interacting with another human being is a challenge at the best of times, which is why we have self-help books, therapists, marriage counsellors, social workers, and liquor stores. But dementia can frequently complicate the process considerably. As the condition progresses, the loved one can exhibit declining precision in speech, disruption of conversational conventions, depression and fear, repeated actions and gestures, or violent agitation for no apparent reason. These symptoms are disorienting for the caregiver, requiring repeated adaptation to new behaviors that require fresh interpretation. The loved one's speech and behavior may make little sense in the real world, but they still require attention and a loving response of some kind.

Mode 3: Advocating

Frye calls this the "rhetorical" or "ideological" mode. I call my version the "advocating" mode. In this mode, we are appealing less to reason than to a sense of "commitment" that precedes reason: an underlying sense of membership in, and belonging to, a group, a cause, or a community. Imagine Shakespeare's Henry V, praising his exhausted soldiers as "We few, we happy few, we band of brothers." Imagine Winston Churchill bracing England for its "finest hour" in the Second World War. Think of Martin Luther King, Jr. sharing his dream on the March to Washington in 1963. Frye distinguishes this mode by a principle "that we belong to something before we are anything, that our loyalties and sense of solidarity are prior to intelligence."[7] In simpler terms, there are times when you've got to look out for your own and to stand up and fight for the people in your care.

When you're caring for a loved one with dementia, you are often surrounded by many voices professing to be on your side. Doctors, nurses, gerontologists, Alzheimer societies, government departments, retirement homes. All of them in their different ways are explicitly dedicated to helping you and your loved one as you navigate the complexities of care. But it doesn't always feel that way. The actions don't always match up with the voices, a fact that erupted into the national consciousness with the COVID crisis and its impact on long-term care facilities. Doctors, nurses, gerontologists, government officials, and retirement home directors have to make difficult and complex decisions. And as personal family caregivers of people we love, we develop a pressing need for a declaration of fundamental loyalty from the people who've been buzzing around us with reassuring words. We want to ask: Beneath all the complexity of empirical fact, and beneath all the logistical demands of providing care to large numbers of people, where is your loyalty? To the person or to the system?

Here we enter the advocating mode: the mode in which we look, not just at the words of those who profess to help us, but at signs that indicate a fundamental commitment that precedes reasoning. And we also ask ourselves this question when negotiating our loyalty to the loved one alongside our loyalties to other ties in our lives – to family, to work, and to ourselves. What is our limit? How far will we go?

Mode 4: Imagining

Frye's fourth mode, which he calls "imaginative," marks a significant shift to a deeper level. In this mode, something that happens in the other modes triggers an awareness of something deeper and more mysterious. A serious diagnosis, for example, or a death in the family might inspire thoughts that we would ordinarily ignore or acknowledge only superficially: mysteries of. birth and death, awareness of the arbitrariness of life, a sense of awe and wonder.[8] George Eliot once called this sensation experiencing "the truth of a commonplace," where the mundane realities of life suddenly take on a new significance. This is the mode, Frye argues, in which we create order through our imaginations, transforming fact, argument, and ideology into a set of narratives that he calls myths.

There's no shortage of mundane reality when you're caring for a family member with dementia. Indeed, those mundane details loom larger and larger as time goes by, and activities such as dressing and personal hygiene, which used to take place behind the scenes, become overt and require planning and deliberation. Nonetheless, when you're sitting with a loved one who is undergoing such drastic transformations in cognition and emotion and behavior, it is difficult to block out those deep questions. Mysteries of birth and death, awareness of the arbitrariness of life, and awe and wonder tend to surface in long and weary vigils, bearing witness to the progress of the disease on the body and mind of someone we love.

So what gets created? We may not have much to do with myths, as Frye imagines, but we do enter new territory: a mode of discourse that appears fitfully in the experiences of caregivers, but which is gaining steady ground in research and practice. It begins in the recognition that creativity, imagination, and skill do not desert individuals completely when dementia strikes: that persons with dementia can continue, not just to enjoy such things as music and dance, but to create music and dance, and that such creativity can serve as powerful mnemonic aids to those with impaired memory. And bearing witness to that creativity, however sporadically it appears, widens our awareness of the loved one, and amplifies our capacity for mutual communication.

These are the four modes I will be using in the chapters that follow. While the authors of the published memoirs touch on all four modes, each has anchors in different places. Heather Menzies brings all her skills as a journalist to bear as she assembles knowledge from different experts and specialists to describe her mother's condition. Mike Barnes gives deep insight into the caregiver's role as an advocate for a loved one, not just when facing the health care system, but in facing dementia itself. Cathie Borrie gives poignant voice to both the understanding mode, as she listens to her mother's conversation, and the imagining mode, as she renders their conversations as a form of lyricism. The ten people I interviewed directly crossed all four modes while describing their experiences of dementia care. They switched hats constantly as the need arose, illuminating an important point: that the same information, the same person, the same experience can belong to more than one mode.

Frye posits that the same text can be interpreted differently according to different prevailing modes of interpretation. Information relating to dementia care has the same fluidity. A person with dementia may eloquently describe a recent trip to Florida to guests who come to visit; only the silent, patient caregiver knows that the loved one has never been to Florida, and that the account, while internally consistent, has absolutely no bearing in reality. The words of a retirement home administrator may seem intelligent, wise, and informed during an introductory tour of the facility, and then woefully hypocritical after the loved one has suffered a serious fall. A caregiver may learn to block out the monotonous tone of a person repeating the same phrase over and over again, and then be startled into attention when the repetitions start to take on a rhythm suggestive of poetry or incantation.

Mode, then, does not lie solely in the mind of the caregiver, nor solely in the mind of the care recipient. Mode is something that happens between the two; it shifts according to the time, the day, the task, the predicament. But for all the uncertainty, I maintain that there are patterns of regularity, familiar grooves. And if we can sort out those regularities, organize them, and understand them more fully, it could alleviate substantially the exhausting ordeal of a caregiver who is wearing so many hats for such a long time.

PART TWO

Getting the Facts

The Describing Mode

The only description of his condition was "cognitive impairment." The neurologist discounted Lewy body, but thought it was more hepatic encephalopathy (HE). The liver doctor felt that he didn't display enough signs for HE and felt it was some form of dementia. Our family doctor describes it as a form of dementia exacerbated by varying episodes of HE. So on we go.

– Participant Jane

CHAPTER THREE

Labelling Dementia

The doctor's expression didn't change. Only her hand moved, pulling the manila folder closer, opening it up: the evidence. The hard, objective evidence.
Instantly I hated her.

– Heather Menzies[1]

Heather Menzies is an author and journalist, awarded the Order of Canada in 2013 in recognition of her "contributions to public discourse." One might add "diverse" to that statement of tribute. Her ten books cover topics ranging from the commons tradition in Scotland to the human costs of globalization, Ontario's cheese industry, the effects of informatics on employment in Canada, and most recently reconciliation with the Indigenous peoples of North America.[2] Among these varied books, not to mention numerous magazine articles, teaching, and speaking engagements, she found time in 2009 to publish *Enter Mourning*, an account of her mother's battle with Alzheimer's disease.

As the adult daughter and primary caregiver of an independent and often stubborn woman, Menzies experienced the full impact of dementia on a family's effort to live in a world of social and physical realities. She witnessed the steady decline of her mother's housekeeping, to the point of nearly setting the home on fire. She weathered accusatory stares from neighbors who noticed the mother's neglect of her dog, and the anxiety of discovering that her mother had lost her way while driving and had to be led home by a kindly stranger. And she endured disagreements among her siblings about the nature and severity of her mother's condition.

In addition to these challenges, Menzies experienced the pain of receiving "hard, objective evidence," however sympathetically conveyed, and the complexity of diagnosing her mother's medical condition, with all the tests and procedures. The doctor, anticipating her confusion, supplied her with information on Alzheimer's disease at the time of diagnosis; like many people, she ignored it at the time.

After her mother's death, however, Menzies, a curious and thoughtful journalist, went to work. She read; she interviewed doctors and researchers and specialists. She wanted to understand, in scientific terms, what her mother had experienced. The quest brought her to learn about neurology, about toxic buildup of beta-amyloids in the hippocampus, about the psychology of memory loss and the science behind articulate speech. She became what's known in medicine as a "lay expert." And she's not alone.

Put two or more personal caregivers in a room together and the terms proliferate. Alzheimer's. Lewy body. Fronto-temporal. Vascular. Ischemic. Sundowning. MOCA test. PSW. Geriatrician. Hospice. Aricept. Ativan. Cognition. Assessment. Primary progressive aphasia. Caring for someone with dementia is a great way to develop lay expertise: knowledge in an area normally governed by trained experts gained not through formal education or training, but through intensive, sustained direct experience.[3] Like many instances of lay expertise, the knowledge of family caregivers can reach levels of accuracy and insight that startle themselves, let alone professionals who assume that the rest of the population lives in ignorance. But their expertise typically has a surgically narrow focus: on the individuals for whom they personally care. And they use this lay expertise to understand and cope with what is happening to their loved ones in terms of the reality that I loosely call "the real world."

The "real world," as I define it, comprises all those features of a normal life that have been rendered strange or unfamiliar to a person living with a cognitive deficit. This external "reality" can be defined on various levels. In the most general sense, the real world encompasses nebulous laws of social life: conventions of behavior and human interaction; regular rhythms of activity such as meal times and sleeping times; maintenance both of order in the home and of personal hygiene. Our first stirrings of worry may be triggered by the loved one's uncharacteristic clothing choices, or an increasing frequency of non-urgent phone calls late at night. By the same token, we may notice that the loved one is approaching normal, everyday tasks with unusual deliberation, or is less able to handle unexpected events, such as a visitor dropping in unannounced.

At a narrower level of focus, we can define the "real world" as all those affordances of daily life that slip beyond a person's grasp. These include such mundane capabilities as reading traffic signs, handling the television remote control, handling tools, operating a microwave, doing taxes, or remembering to turn off the stove. At this level, the caregiver watches the loved one carefully for indications that an important change has become necessary: accepting home care, surrendering the car keys, or moving into assisted living.

On a still narrower level, the real world consists of the various ways in which the care process itself impinges on the person's life: interactions with doctors, gerontologists, support workers, pharmacists and care network administrators; managing complex medications; submitting to multiple physical and mental examinations. When you find yourself thinking and planning for someone besides yourself, and that person has significant needs, your life can easily become a spreadsheet with hundreds of rows and hundreds of columns, with each cell containing something you have to do to satisfy the world out there.

And finally, we can narrow the real world down to the world of physical laws, represented by bodies of scientific and medical empirical knowledge. This is the level of medical research, medical diagnoses, and medical treatments. Here is where the caregiver and the loved one together engage in the most intense and concentrated effort to understand, in real-world terms, what is happening and what can be done. What is causing the changes we are witnessing? And how can we respond? What treatments are available? What services are available? What decisions lie ahead? How much time do we have? In the face of baffling and frightening internal changes, we look to the medical establishment to explain the experience in real-world terms.

The Descriptive Mode: What Is Happening?

As the mediator between the person with dementia and the real world, the caregiver faces an onslaught of information in the descriptive mode: guidebooks, instruction manuals, government regulations, and information websites. They instruct the caregiver on financial and legal arrangements; home care and assisted living options; medication and nutrition; specialist appointments; directions to various hospitals, clinics, community centers, and hospices.

And yet when Heather Menzies's mother was diagnosed, Menzies used every excuse she could "to ignore the literature on Alzheimer's that the doctor had given us, ignoring what it had to teach us."[4] Only later was she ready to read it and follow it up. Why?

I want to suggest that in dementia caregiving, particularly in the early stages, the real world can often be a frightening, censorious, and implacable eye that we want to avoid. In those early days of forgotten words, burned toast, strange phone calls, and conversational non sequiturs, the possibility that there may be something "wrong" sits like the proverbial elephant in the room. Family members become nervously aware of the curious eyes of neighbors; the tactful care with which the kindly cashier at the local store helps the loved one count out her money; the awkward probing of friends who have clearly noticed something odd.

In resistance to those questioning eyes of the world around us, we may turn inward for a time, explaining what we observe in terms of the loved one's eccentricity: charming foibles that have caused us to shake our heads in resignation for years. "Well, that's your mother, you know. She's always had her head in the clouds." "That's just Dad being Dad." But sooner or later, willingly or unwillingly, our eyes turn outward to that formidable manila folder on the doctor's desk: the one that contains the "hard, objective evidence" that aroused such hostility for Menzies.

In the descriptive mode, we decide, often after a bitter inner struggle, to turn our gaze outward. We face the people – doctors, gerontologists, specialists – who represent empirical science and modern medicine and ask, what is my loved one's condition? What is causing this condition? How is it progressing? And what can I expect in the future? These questions arise with great force at the time of diagnosis: the time when one or more medical experts define and explain the loved one's condition in terms of medicine, science, and empirical reality as we can best understand it. For the remainder of this chapter and the next, I will be focusing on the practice of diagnosing dementia.

Definition

Let's begin with some formal definitions. *Stedman's Medical Dictionary* (2006) defines dementia as

> the loss, usually progressive, of cognitive and intellectual functions, without impairment of perception or consciousness; caused by a variety of disorders, (structural or degenerative) but most commonly associated with structural brain disease. Characterized by disorientation, impaired memory, judgment, and intellect, and a shallow labile affect.[5]

There's a lot in that definition, and it's worth enumerating what we can expect:

- *Loss*: of the loved one's ability to think and capacity to learn. What's more, we can't blame it on either unconsciousness, or deafness, or blindness, or any other kind of impaired sense. Your loved one could be wide awake and able to hear and see as well as ever, and yet suffer loss.
- *More loss:* yes, it gets worse. Dementia is not a one-time event.

- *Multiple causes:* there are many possibilities, most of them related to the brain.
- Common features:

  - *Disorientation*: we can expect confusion, and along with confusion we can expect fear
  - *Mental impairment*: loss of memory; loss of judgment; loss of intellect
  - *Emotional impairment*: unexpected, sometimes inappropriate emotional responses

Other definitions echo Stedman. The fifth edition of the *Diagnostic and Statistics Manual* (*DSM*) defines dementia not as a disease but as a "cluster of neurological disorders ... characterized by the presence of cognitive deficits that are the most prominent and defining features of a given condition."[6] The American Academy of Family Physicians likewise defines dementia as "a group of symptoms that can be caused by brain damage."[7] The National Library of Medicine's Medline Plus defines it as "a loss of mental functions severe enough to affect your daily life and activities."[8] The National Institute of Neurological Disorders and Stroke also emphasizes "the loss of cognitive functioning ... [that] interferes with a person's daily life and activities."[9] Out of these various definitions and the surrounding explanations provided by these sources, several points are worth nothing.

Symptom vs. Cause

First, the medical research community makes a distinction between *symptom* and *cause* (also termed *etiology*). "Dementia" as a term refers to a group of symptoms; these symptoms are caused by an underlying disease or disorder. To say that a loved one has "dementia," then, is not like saying the loved one has cancer or diabetes. Rather, the loved one suffers from one or more diseases or injuries, which have caused one or more cognitive deficits.

According to the Alzheimer's Association, Alzheimer's Disease accounts for 60–80 per cent of dementia cases, which is why so many support services for dementia come from societies calling themselves "Alzheimer's associations."[10] But this can cause some confusion: Alzheimer's disease is a specific disease, and thus one of the various causes of dementia. But the term "Alzheimer's" has also come to be used as a general synonym for dementia. And if we're using the term that way, it means that we're describing not a disease but a set of symptoms.

What's the Actual Cause?

Second, the manifestations of dementia can arise from a wide range of causes. Symptoms of Alzheimer's disease are similar to those of other causes such as Lewy body or frontotemporal dementia. They can also arise from causes beyond dementia, as side effects of other problems such as drug use, poor nutrition, depression, or an infection that causes disorientation.[11] This has led to a persistent concern regarding misdiagnosis, in both research and practice. And clinicians can easily confuse one kind of dementia with another, or with another condition altogether. Such confusion can easily delay crucial diagnosis, particularly in cases of early onset dementia, as well as administration of inappropriate therapies and medications.

Normal vs. Abnormal

Finally, medical sources agree: dementia is not to be confused with the "normal" decline of human capacity that awaits all of us who live long enough. Dementia is "not related to normal aging," declares the American Academy of Family Physicians.[12] "While everyone loses some neurons as they age," advises the National Institute for Neurological Disorders and Strokes, "people with dementia experience far greater loss. Unlike dementia, age-related memory loss isn't disabling."[13] The National Library of Medicine concurs: "It is normal to become a bit more forgetful as you age. But dementia is not a normal part of aging."[14]

For Menzies and her mother, as for all those I interviewed, and for everyone who reluctantly brings a frightened and confused relative to a medical professional for answers, the diagnostic experience marks the intersection of two different destinies. A person who doesn't have dementia will die eventually, but "normally." A person with a form of dementia such as Alzheimer's will die eventually, but "abnormally." The key difference, it seems, lies in that term "disabling," and the emphasis placed by the National Institute of Neurological Disorders and Stroke on "interference with a person's daily life and activities." Without dementia, we will hopefully retain some measure of control over our lives, together with the power to make our own choices and decisions. With dementia, we will probably die in a state of complete helplessness.

In this sense, a diagnosis of dementia – and, indeed, the descriptive mode as a whole – can feel like a curse. However gently and tactfully a doctor might open that manila folder and relay the "hard, cold evidence," it can feel like a sentence from above that descends, seemingly at random, upon the loved one, wreaking havoc on the life of the entire family. To make matters worse, a family rarely has a clear notion of the cause, or of what the person might or might not have done in the past to avoid it.

Given this distressing state of affairs, it is small wonder that the medical community is struggling to mitigate the devastating impact of a dementia diagnosis. And part of that struggle is located in small but significant changes to the words it uses to define and describe it.

Vocabulary

If we venture outside the confines of medical practice, we find that the term "dementia" raises some problems. According to the *Oxford English Dictionary* (2013), the word has historically signified "insanity," and the historical instances of usage paint a grim picture. A citation from 1806 distinguishes dementia from "curable mania" and equates it with "idiotism." The OED also lists a more general definition: "Complete loss of judgement; (wild) foolishness resembling insanity." The OED cites a usage of this definition as late as 2010: "It was when I switched on the news yesterday ... that I knew for sure we are in the grip of collective dementia." "Dementia" as a term carries historical connotations of insanity in its wildest manifestations. Think of the mysterious figure in Charlotte Bronte's *Jane Eyre*, hidden in the attic, cackling with eerie laughter in the dead of night, ferociously attacking others, and eventually burning down the house and jumping to her death. Think of the "dementors" in the Harry Potter books, assailing the students at Hogwarts with the power to generate despair.[15] These are not images we care to associate with someone we love, nor do we take kindly to the idea of locking that person up as a guilty secret, someone to be restrained, guarded, and hidden from everyday society.

If that particular OED usage emphasizes the violence of insanity, the Library of Congress, in its list of standard subject headings for its library catalogue, links dementia to old age. Certain kinds of dementia, including Alzheimer's disease, are related not directly to dementia, but to a narrower term: **Senile dementia**.

The OED defines "senile" as "pertaining to old age," and senile dementia as "a severe form of senile deterioration." A cited usage from 1948 argues that "the senile dement exhibits to a profound degree the characteristic failings of the deteriorated senile persons." Dementia, in its most common forms, is thus associated primarily with old age, and a particularly humiliating vision of old age. Senile dementia, in this vision, is a more intense and extreme version of what awaits us all in the final stage of Shakespeare's "Ages" speech in *As You Like It*: "second childishness and mere oblivion: sans teeth, sans eyes, sans taste, sans everything."

Given these associations, we can well understand why many families are reluctant to face the evidence until it becomes necessary. And it is hardly surprising that the fifth edition of the *DSM* has changed its terms. While it retains the word "dementia" parenthetically, the *DSM-5* now favors the term **Major Neurocognitive Disorder**. The change has two important purposes. First, it loosens, to some degree, the tight association of dementia with old age. Both research and clinical communities have much to learn about early onset forms of dementia, and changing the term will hopefully make it easier to identify and study instances of dementia among younger people.

Second, the term "major neurocognitive disorder" aims to gain some clinical and terminological distance from the frightening and disparaging associations that adhere to the word "dementia" and its unwitting suggestion that a dearly loved parent or spouse is going to go wildly and destructively insane before collapsing into "second childishness." Behavioral changes may well occur, as may unwitting damage; helplessness does indeed lie ahead. But the new term will hopefully make conceptual room for a broader range of consequences and with less social stigma.

"Major Neurocognitive Disorder" is an unwieldy term, to be sure, which is partly why I have elected to continue using the term "dementia" in my own research, despite its unfortunate connotations. Nonetheless, the advent of this new term in *DSM-5* provides an example of how a terminological shift can effect a change in thinking and assumptions.

The Story So Far

This chapter leaves us with bad news and good news.

First, the bad news. Approaching dementia from the perspective of the descriptive mode, defining it in terms of the world of science and medicine, leads us into a labyrinth of complexity. We're not dealing with a disease so much as a set of symptoms that could come from any number of sources. For all the precision of medical terminology and the rigor of the scientific method, there are many opportunities to get things wrong. And hovering over it all lies that bleak insistence: dementia is not normal. Your loved one has pulled the short straw, and no one can say why or whether different behaviors in the past might have made any difference.

Now for the good news. This isn't *Jane Eyre*. Nor is it Hogwarts. When we step into a doctor's office and open that manila folder, we're no longer in the world of novels, with their capacity for generating terror by tapping into our unnamed fears. We're dealing with something real. It has names. It has definitions. It has boundaries.

And as Menzies later discovered, it's actually very, very interesting. It's also inspiring. There are hosts of intelligent and accomplished researchers and practitioners working on this: neurologists, psychologists, speech therapists, artists, musicians, computer programmers, architects, social workers, librarians, philosophers, politicians. In their different ways, they are endeavoring, with patience and persistence, to understand dementia, to explain it, to treat it, and one day hopefully to cure it. Indeed, we'll continue drawing on such research in the later chapters.

Addressing dementia in the real world of empirical fact, honest research, and shared knowledge helps us to see dementia, and personal dementia care, not as a private disgrace, but as a shared community challenge. It might not be the challenge we would have chosen, but if that's where we've landed, at least we're not facing it alone.

But yes, as a medical condition, dementia is very confusing. And to deal with it, we need to do a bit more work. In the next chapter, we'll look at how our medical and psychological understanding of dementia is organized. And further possibilities will open up.

CHAPTER FOUR

Classifying Dementia

Classification I: The Disciplinary Roots

If you're searching for information on dementia in the descriptive mode, you may well find yourself searching MEDLINE: a massive database maintained by the United States National Library of Medicine, which contains over 31 million references to journal articles in the life sciences.[1] That's a daunting number, and few of us feel inclined to spend a lot of time reading all those articles, even if we could understand their specialized languages and advanced research methods. But there's something interesting about the way they're organized.

The NLM indexes these articles using an elaborate system of headings known as "MeSH," short for *Medical Subject Headings*. These headings are carefully classified into different categories, and you may be surprised to find that within the MeSH headings, "dementia" appears twice: as a **Mental Disorder (F03)** and as a **Nervous System Disease (C10)**. A mental disorder, according to MeSH, is an illness or disease that causes "abnormalities of thought, feeling and behavior producing either distress or impairment of function" (MeSH F03). Nervous system diseases, according to MeSH, are "disorders of the brain, spinal cord, cranial nerves, peripheral nerves, nerve roots, autonomic nervous system, neuromuscular junction and muscle" (MeSH C10).[2]

These two definitions speak to a strange characteristic of dementia as a neurocognitive disorder. The condition derives its definition from two related but distinct areas of research: psychology and neurology. If psychology addresses thought, neuropsychology addresses the brain. We define and classify mental disorders by their thoughts, and we identify those thoughts by their symptoms. Nervous system diseases, by contrast, are defined by their causes: malfunctions in the brain that we can hopefully identify and measure. The neurological approach, therefore, aims for the detection and measurement of source causes, while the broader psychological approach aims for precise and accurate measurement of symptoms, followed by careful inference as to the cause.

Neurological Approaches

As with cancer research, dementia research maintains a strong focus on biomarkers: molecules found in blood, tissues, or body fluids that signify the presence or absence of a condition or disease.[3] Indeed, there's been some progress on that front. Gene codings, for instance, provide some evidence of frontotemporal dementia, and MRI or CT scans can suggest the presence of vascular dementia. It's amazing what science and technology can do nowadays.

Unfortunately, at the time of this writing, biomarkers are too preliminary to be very useful for clinical diagnosis, even for those who have mastered all the science and its accompanying acronyms. While patterns of genetic mutation are undoubtedly a fruitful avenue of research, and while they may increase the strength of a diagnosis based on clinical assessment, the NIA-AA guidelines on Alzheimer's disease diagnosis do not recommend their use for routine diagnostic purposes. Such tests need greater standardization in their design and in their interpretation. Furthermore, not all communities have access to them. And besides, if you're looking for a simple yes or no, biomarker tests can be just as frustrating as all the other diagnostic methods. According to the NIA-AA, biomarker results fall into three categories: "clearly positive, clearly negative, and indeterminate."[4] Neurological approaches, for all their commitment to precise measurement, can still drop us off in the land of "maybe."

Cognitive Approaches

Cognitive approaches, being concerned with thoughts and behaviors, probably make more immediate sense to the caregiver. The *DSM-5*[5] enumerates six distinct domains of cognition, each of which expresses a different facet of thinking and reasoning.[6] Perhaps the most obvious, and most immediately associated with dementia, are the following:

- *Language*: the ease and fluency with which we can name objects and use words with correct grammar and syntax.
- *Learning and Memory*: our ability to remember names and events, with or without cues, and to recognize places, objects, and people, both in the short and long terms.

Searching for words and searching for memories. As a caregiver you'll probably spend a lot of time seeing your loved one hunting for one or both. And whether the words are hiding or the memories have disappeared, the floundering and confusion can appear much the same in both cases.

Other domains are especially vulnerable to misdiagnosis:

- *Perceptual-Motor Function*: our ability to perceive and visually interpret our environment, as well as retain our perceptual motor coordination. Symptoms of decline might include impaired sense of direction or inability to interpret familiar landmarks, or unusual patterns of walking. Such symptoms can easily be confused with delirium, head trauma, hydrocephalus, or problems with hearing or vision.[7] When Participant Victor visited his father in the hospital after his fall, he couldn't tell if his father was suffering from dementia, from the effects of his fall, or from hospital psychosis. He only knew that his father was seeing insects crawling up the hospital walls.
- *Social Cognition*: our capacity to feel and recognize emotions and to have insights. Decline in this domain can easily resemble clinical depression.

Two other domains can be particularly cryptic:

- *Complex Attention*: our capacity to sustain attention and pay selective attention when in crowded or noisy environments. This can be difficult to detect, especially in people who are natural introverts; one hardly needs to have dementia to find the clamor of modern social stimuli overwhelming.
- *Executive Function*: our ability to plan, decide, and respond to others with flexibility and reasonable restraint. These symptoms can easily be obscured, particularly in parent-child

relationships, by the adult child's habitual tendency to trust and defer to figures of security and authority. As Participant Mary stated, it was very easy to trust her father, who had been a tax lawyer for years, when he assured her that he had his taxes well in hand. As it turned out, he didn't, and hadn't for some time.

The *DSM-5* defines a neurocognitive disorder, minor or major, as "a clear decline from a previous level of functioning in one or more of the key cognitive domains."[8] If we reframe the *DSM-5*'s six domains as verbs rather than nouns, the human mind emerges as a complex balance of six primary activities:

- Speaking
- Remembering
- Seeing
- Listening
- Understanding
- Responding

What is more, each of these verbs refers implicitly to the world of lived reality. Is the loved one saying things that make sense and remembering things that actually happened? Does the person see or hear what is actually there? Does the person understand what is happening in the surrounding environment and respond to it in an appropriate manner?

Dementia, then, can be defined as a disruption in a delicate network of methods whereby our minds interact with the real world. And what makes it "dementia," as we understand it, is the degree to which the disruption impairs our ability to interact with the outside world on a daily basis.

Classification II: The Diagnosis

Having established this background, let's examine the process of diagnosis as defined by the *DSM-5*. As we'll see, a diagnosis of dementia comes after a complex chain of tests and inferences.

To be diagnosed with dementia, the person in your care must exhibit a decline in at least one of the six cognitive domains, and the evidence must result from the following:

- an expressed concern, directly from your loved one, from the clinician, or from a concerned individual such as yourself: a family member or other experienced caregiver;
- a clinical assessment, preferably based on some standard neurocognitive assessment, such as the Montreal Cognitive Assessment (MoCA).

Upon establishing such evidence, the doctor must then eliminate possible other causes, by ensuring:

- that the symptoms do not occur only in the context of delirium. We can see and say and do a lot of eccentric things when recovering from surgery, suffering from a high temperature or reacting badly to medication.[9] But when the temperature goes down and the meds get sorted out, do the symptoms persist? Or do they go away?
- that no other mental disorder would provide a better explanation of the symptoms.

If other causes have been eliminated, the doctor would determine that the patient is exhibiting the symptoms of a neurocognitive disorder. We are now in dementia territory.

Having made this determination, the clinician must then categorize it as "major" or "minor," with "major neurocognitive disorder" meaning "dementia" and "minor neurocognitive disorder" meaning a much milder condition that may or may not develop into dementia. This classification involves two distinct factors:

- the degree of impairment: "modest" in the case of minor neurocognitive disorder, and "significant" and "substantial" in the case of major neurocognitive disorder;
- the degree of interference in the activities of daily life.

This can be rather a poser. How exactly do we measure the interference in daily activities? Daily life is different for all of us; the world places different demands on different people in different situations. And even at our brightest, most of us have been guilty of losing our phones, locking ourselves out of the house, or leaving our belongings behind on the bus. At what point do we draw the line between a "modest" impairment and a "significant" impairment? "Dementia," then, is defined as a crucial increase in intensity and disruptiveness. We started with a grim "yes/no" question: Sick or well? Normal or abnormal? We now find that answer lies along a continuous line, with markers inserted: "normal," "minor neurocognitive disorder," and "major cognitive disorder."

Let's assume that the clinician has determined the presence of a major neurocognitive disorder. As a next step, the clinician proceeds to classify it as one or more subtypes, such as Alzheimer's disease, Lewy body syndrome, or vascular dementia. The *DSM-5* enumerates ten specific sub-types of dementia, along with categories for "other," "multiple," and "unspecified." Categorizing the disorder into one of these categories requires an analysis of the symptoms, together with a listing of potential causative factors.[10]

A diagnosis of Alzheimer's disease, for instance, requires evidence of decline in at least two cognitive domains, one of which must be learning and memory. Decline in learning and memory alone is sufficient for a diagnosis of Alzheimer's disease, provided that the pattern shows insidious onset and gradual progression. A diagnosis of Lewy body disease, by contrast, requires evidence of changes in complex attention and executive function. The *DSM-5* lists a set of "core features" and another of "suggestive features" related to Lewy body disease, and a diagnosis of Lewy body disease requires evidence of either two core features, or one core feature and one or more suggestive features.[11]

Once again, the diagnostic process is a complex and uncertain one. Some forms of dementia, such as Parkinson's or Huntington's disease, exhibit evidence from the first onset of symptoms. With others, such as Alzheimer's, the symptoms appear first, and the causes reveal themselves only slowly over time. Furthermore, the patient could be suffering from multiple disorders: what participant Jane referred to wearily as "co-morbidities abounding." Finally, none of the diagnostic criteria professes to be definite. Certain criteria can only be termed definite through evidence of autopsy.

Medical researchers are struggling to change this, and in recent years, they have even turned to algorithms, similar to those that govern our streaming and social media sites. Given modern computing ability to analyze large quantities of data for suggestive patterns that could yield useful insights, perhaps such data analysis could be used in the diagnosis and treatment of dementia.[12] As with biomarkers, however, the contribution of algorithmic methods of dementia prediction and diagnosis are yet to be firmly established at this time of writing. While the increased power of current computing may enable us to provide more precise measurement of different phenomena, it has not, as yet, offered us any substantial improvement of, or alternative to, current diagnostic practice.

Vocabulary and Classification: The Story So Far

Where are we, then, after bringing someone in for a clinical assessment and receiving a diagnosis of dementia? This assessment, if performed carefully and conscientiously, is an impressive reasoning process, involving multiple stages of classification and elimination. The clinician has performed a series of standard tests and has categorized the results carefully. Possible non-dementia causes have been eliminated; the extent of the cognitive deficit is great enough to characterize it as a major neurocognitive disorder; the dementia is affecting at least one of six primary cognitive domains and that it can be tentatively attributed to one or more etiological subtypes.

In the process, you as the caregiver have probably acquired some impressive lay expertise, particularly if the clinician is willing to explain the diagnostic process as it proceeds. You have confronted a range of names that may not have been in your initial vocabulary: perceptual-motor coordination, semantic memory, executive function, neurocognitive disorder, fronto-temporal lobar degeneration, ischaemic lesions, cerebral microbleeds, hyperorality, progressive aphasia. The disorder which may have rested in dread silence has finally surfaced. But instead of being dressed in colloquial euphemisms – "troubling," "struggling," "having a rough time," "you don't suppose," or "let's not go there just now" – dementia emerges clad in the vocabulary of the descriptive mode of psychology and neuropsychology:

vocabulary that attempts to describe a real-world phenomenon as accurately and precisely as possible.

Nonetheless, while you as the caregiver may be feeling greater agency by the knowledge you're gaining, the clinician may be experiencing the reverse. Because underneath all of this careful and rigorous reasoning lies a deeply frustrating reality. No matter how much we know about disruption of the neural substrates, a diagnosis of dementia comes down to human judgment. The *DSM-5* is at pains to point out that the diagnosis of a major neurocognitive disorder "relies on an insightful report by the individual and/or a family member, and a level of good judgement from the clinician."[13] Likewise, the National Institue on Aging: Alzheimer Associations (NIA-AA) guidelines emphasize that diagnosis is "inherently a clinical judgment made by a skilled clinician."[14] Diagnosing your loved one's dementia, it seems, is a "judgment call," derived from ambiguous data and the caregiver's subjective and inexpert expressions of concern.

So the uncertainty continues, along with the worry and the questions. When we take our loved one in for clinical assessment, we are appealing to the guardians and representatives of the descriptive mode, in the form of clinical practice, in order to answer an important and frightening question: is this person for whom I deeply care suffering from an abnormal condition of aging that will overturn both our lives and end in death? This appears to be a yes or no question: a frightening binarism requiring a one-word answer. But it isn't. The answer could be "yes," it could be "no," and it could also be "maybe."

In such cases, the questions and the worry and the uncertainty may lead us to reject the descriptive mode altogether and to rail against a medical system that appears vague, noncommittal, and unhelpful. But even at its most frustrating junctures, the methods and categories of the descriptive mode – dementia as defined and conceived in conventional medicine – there are important things we can learn.

Qualitative vs. Quantitative Measurement

If, as the *DSM-5* and NIA-AA both agree, a good diagnosis rests on good judgment, then you as the caregiver remain intimately involved. While the clinician's judgment relies partly on standardized cognitive tests such as drawing the hands of a clock, it also rests heavily upon the evidence of changes in the person's capabilities and behavior. And in such cases, the caregiver is essential for helping the loved one supply information regarding the timing of events and the nature of the symptoms. Long-term, intimate knowledge of the patient's nature, habits, and capabilities enables the caregiver and help the clinician determine what constitutes significant changes in the six cognitive domains. As the clinician talks to the patient in the presence of the caregiver, long experience of the loved one enables the caregiver to recognize irrelevant or flippant remarks, not necessarily as dementia, but as manifestations of anxiety and fear. In any condition with insidious onset, the close observation of someone onsite, with accurate and intimate knowledge, becomes essential. In any condition brought about by a specific event, such as a stroke, the caregiver can provide important details about the symptoms and the time of onset. However frustrated and impatient you may become through the diagnostic process, your insights and your contributions remain deeply necessary.

Binary Divisions vs. Continuous Variables

Part of the ambiguity inherent in dementia diagnoses – an ambiguity that requires the judgment I mention – lies in the fact that with dementia we are imposing categorical distinctions upon an inherently continuous spectrum. According to the *DSM-5*, "Mild and major neurocognitive disorders are categorical diagnostic constructs imposed on an underlying continuum of cognitive impairment from normality to severe impairment, as seen in the clinic and the population."[15] In other words, doctors may classify you, but they don't put you in a cage: rather, they place you at a certain place along a continuous line.

And here's an added complexity. Just because you're on a continuous line doesn't mean that you're inevitably moving along it like a train. The presence of a mild cognitive impairment provides no guarantee that a major impairment will follow, and the presence of significant genetic markers does not decree that the person will develop dementia in the future. Indeed, the *DSM-5*'s new category of "mild neurocognitive disorder" has prompted resistance in some areas, arguing that it might lead to large numbers of persons unnecessarily concerned, "leading to unnecessary diagnostic tests and unproven treatments."[16]

Medical Context vs. Social Context

Finally, in the case of dementia diagnosis, we have to acknowledge that the "real world," as I call it in the descriptive mode, is not just a matter of physics, chemistry, and biology; nor is it confined to the terms and methods and procedures of applied sciences like medicine. The real world also includes our social reality: our laws, our traditions, our communities, our languages, our shared beliefs. Physical laws exist alongside social patterns. And in dementia diagnosis, the physical and the social are intricately and awkwardly intertwined. Definitions of dementia, whatever the cause, keep circling back to this notion of "interference in daily life."

On the one hand, standards such as the International Classification of Diseases (ICD; 2019) warn us against overreliance on social indicators of performance in a diagnosis: "Changes in role performance, such as lowered ability to keep or find a job, should not be used as a criteria of dementia, because of the large cross-cultural differences that exist in what is appropriate, and because there may be frequent, externally-imposed changes in the availability of work within a given culture."[17]

At the same time, the ICD defines dementia in terms of daily living – "washing, dressing, eating, personal hygiene, excretory and toilet activities" – while noting that "how [decline] manifests itself will depend largely on the social and cultural setting in which the patient lives." The NIA-AA standards define dementia as a condition whose symptoms "interfere with the ability to function at work or at usual activities."[18] And the *DSM-5* distinguishes mild from major neurocognitive disorder according to the disruption accorded to the activities of daily living, such as "paying bills or managing medications."[19]

Social contexts and social procedures lie at the heart of the definition of dementia in the descriptive mode. While the procedures themselves may differ from context to context – not everyone has to balance a checkbook; not everyone cooks dinner every day – their performance or nonperformance largely determine a diagnosis of dementia or major neurocognitive disorder. Whatever may be going on in the brain is intricately and inextricably linked to the person's life in the world: at home, at work, in the community, with friends, with family, and even alone.

Conclusion

What are we to make, then, of the descriptive mode of information, as manifested by the procedures for diagnosing dementia?

It's a sad and frightening experience, both for you as the caregiver and for the person you're trying to shelter and protect. Clinical findings, test results, and medical definitions can have a hard, cruel edge, as Heather Menzies describes in her memoir. But sooner or later, we have to open that implacable manila folder and examine the evidence. What do we gain from our efforts, and those of the medical community, to define what is happening as a phenomenon in the physical and social world in which we live?

I would argue that we gain, first and foremost, lay expertise. We can't help learning, and however great our resistance, new words, new definitions, and new concepts start to shape our thinking. Monsters conjured up by culturally inherited images of madness and insanity are coaxed out from under our beds and replaced with real-world problems. Life may be as uncertain as ever, but we find ourselves handling it with a greater, more powerful arsenal of words and concepts and strategies.

Make no mistake: as we gain a greater grasp of the ambiguities and mysteries that surround dementia, the problems that lie ahead don't fade away. Rather, they assume a greater and sometimes ruthless clarity. Dementia is irreversible. It lasts a long time. It gets worse. It's terminal. A dementia diagnosis is bad news, to be sure. But in the process of arriving at it – the process of systematically eliminating other possibilities and of categorizing the symptoms to infer the type of dementia involved – we find ourselves moving away from the sense of being cursed. The terrible binary question of "Yes or No" yields to more nuanced questions of degree: "How much?" "How bad?" "How significant?" "How serious?"

Above all, the process of diagnosing dementia, rooted as it is in the descriptive mode of empirical medical practice, forces us as caregivers to recognize the importance of questions that lie beyond the scope of such practice. If we accept the definition of dementia provided by the International Classification of Disease as a condition that disrupts a person's daily living, we need to recognize that daily living is more than simply washing, dressing, and personal hygiene. Caring for a family member with dementia demands far more than an understanding of the phenomenon in terms of pathology and medicine. It demands an understanding of how the family member lives: that ineffable quality that Heidegger called "being-in-the-world." We won't get there just with the *DSM*, and we can't expect our doctors and clinicians to grasp such nuances on their own.

As a family caregiver, you provide a crucial link between the broader care community and the personal life of the person in your care. You know your loved one's personality, habits, values, preferences, and fears. You recognize characteristic and uncharacteristic responses to situations. Above all, as a family caregiver, you have the opportunity to watch and listen to the person you love for extended periods. This is immensely useful for charting the progress of the loved one's condition, and for interpreting evidence that would be mysterious to others. But to do so requires a different mode.

PART THREE

Following the Thread

The Understanding Mode

*You speak a language that I understand not;
My life stands in the level of your dreams.*
— Shakespeare, *The Winter's Tale*,
III.ii, 85–86

CHAPTER FIVE

Conversation

"What does sorrow look like?"
"It's a form of sadness brought about on a gray and heavy day. I've reached the ultimate of the intimate and that's the end of it."
"Oh dear ... Let me ask you, what do you think is the ugliest thing in the world?"
"A lack of dignity. Is that the right answer?"
"Yes. Okay, what about this one: what's the worst thing a person could do to another person?"
"They could throw their sublime into the ridiculous."
"What is so scary about dying?"
"Have you ever tried it?"
"Good point."

– Cathie Borrie in conversation with her mother, *The Long Hello*[1]

Canadian author Cathie Borrie trained as a nurse and holds degrees in both public health and law. Her life has had its share of stresses and complexities: her brother died a violent death at age 13; her mother separated from her alcoholic husband when Borrie was a child; Borrie had a complex and vexed relationship with both her mother and her stepfather during the loneliness of growing up. And when her mother developed Alzheimer's disease, Borrie served as her primary caregiver for seven years, a process which found her reliving a lot of those experiences all over again.

Borrie's account of the experience, *The Long Hello*, describes in selective but precise detail the experience of caregiving, interspersed with recollections of her own life, and her relationship with her mother through her years of growing up. She weaves the two strands together in a rhythmic fashion that resembles the movements of the dance classes she attends as a stress reliever. With regular alternations between past and present, between thoughtful recollections of the past and accounts of conversations and tasks in the present, Borrie evokes the complex and varied sensations of bearing witness to the gradual end of her mother's life.

In the seven years of caregiving, Borrie sat and talked with her mother, listening to her carefully. She also recorded the conversations, and their interchanges form the lyrical core of a story that captures her efforts to understand her mother and her mother's condition, not simply in terms of the outer world of her training in nursing and health and law, but also in terms of her mother's inner world, a world that became more remote as her mother's ability to interact with the outer world gradually lessened. These conversations exemplify what I call the "understanding" mode, roughly analogous to Northrop Frye's conception in *Words with Power* of the "conceptual" or "dialectic" mode.

When Frye referred to the conceptual/dialectic mode, he was thinking of philosophical reasoning: scrutinizing someone's discourse in terms of its internal logic and consistency. He might well be startled, if not horrified, to see me drawing a connection between his conceptual/dialectic mode and my "understanding" mode. After all, the cognitive changes that dementia brings about frequently give rise to behavior and speech that defy logic and consistency, and even sense. All this talk about "throwing the sublime into the ridiculous" may be charming in its way, but I'm not sure Borrie's mother would hold her own in a philosophical debate with Socrates or Bertrand Russell.

Nonetheless, I do make that connection, and what's more, I insist upon it: that to care in a meaningful way for someone with dementia, we need to reach across to understand the situation internally as well as externally, and to retain our capacity to communicate with our loved ones for as long as possible. Above all, we need to remember the words of Dr. Jennifer Bute, a retired doctor who is living with dementia herself:

> Every communication has a purpose, the challenge is to discover it. No word or action is meaningless, what sounds like nonsense or repetition of the same question or sentence are, to express a feeling, to show a need, to give information or to get a response. What appears to be an inappropriate response or action may be a form of communication.[2]

However well the outer world defines the situation in terms of medicine and social services and law, we need to keep listening and observing and interacting with the loved one and try to understand as best we can.

From the Outer World to the Inner World

So far, we've been in the Describing Mode, and thus dealing with the real world: recognizing that our loved one's condition has become "abnormal" in medical terms, as well as in social and legal terms. Caregivers, however, have to split their time between the everyday world we all inhabit and the inner world of the person with dementia. In the early stages, this can be a collaborative exercise, as caregiver and care recipient "negotiate and co-construct an account of their situation."[3] The caregiver might support unobtrusively the efforts of the loved one to retain connections, rather like the two assistants in *The Devil Wears Prada*, tagging discreetly behind Meryl Streep at cocktail parties and whispering the names of the people she meets in her ear. The caregiver can assume a variety of "supporting roles" – secretary, consultant, chauffeur – to help the person organize medications or drive the person to family dinners, shopping trips, and community activities.

As the dementia progresses, this collaboration acquires a nonverbal character, as the caregiver learns to recognize and interpret the gestures that signal the persistence of identity and personality and continuing communicative need.[4] Furthermore, as the outside world becomes stranger and more frightening to the loved one, caregivers take on more and more of the heavy lifting, shifting in the process to a more dominant and overt role. They explain their surroundings to a bewildered person who can no longer recognize a doctor's waiting room. They ensure that rents and expenses are paid; that the loved one appears punctually for appointments; that home care services are in place and working adequately. More painfully, they sometimes need to explain a loved one's aggressive or antisocial behavior to friends, to wait staff, to cashiers, to bus drivers.

To maintain this collaboration requires sympathy, respect, patience, and particularly background knowledge, enabling the caregiver to draw from the person's experience to recognize connections. Family caregivers serve as archives of a shared past, and their close knowledge of the loved one's character and personal history can be very important in understanding how the world looks to the person with dementia. Here's an example.

When Victor visited his father in the family home, he found his father at the kitchen table, with his medication spread out over the table, trying to make sense of which pill was which and when he should take each. Victor sat with his father and sorted out his medication and loaded the pill dispenser accurately with the meds to be taken in the morning and those in the evening. The following day, when he went to visit, he found the pills scattered once again across the kitchen table and his father once again laboriously trying to determine what he was supposed to take and when.

As a measure of the disjunction between normal cognition and a state of dementia, the incident was useful; it certainly served to alert Victor that his father's condition had progressed significantly. The incident, however, could support various interpretations: the father's dismantling of the pill dispenser could have been seen as a sign of rebellion, of frustration, of childish pique. Victor, however, knew that his father had spent his entire life building mechanisms and trouble-shooting machinery. All his life, he had witnessed his father's response to a problem: break the problem into pieces, go right back to first principles, and start again, this time with no mistakes.

For Victor, the incident was frustrating, but hardly surprising. While his father's condition prevented him from resolving his confusion, it had not eroded his central character; what an external observer might have seen as personality change, Victor perceived as something entirely consistent with the man he had known all his life. Beneath all the confusion caused by the cognitive disorder, his dad was still his dad.

Some researchers have taken to calling this ongoing task of collaboration "curation," a term common in information and museum studies, which the *Oxford English Dictionary* defines as "to look after and preserve (the exhibits in a collection, as in a museum); to be the keeper or custodian of (a collection, museum, public garden, etc.)." The caregiver is curating the self-identity of the care recipient, drawing on a deep connection together with background knowledge to maintain and preserve the person's rights, dignity, and entitlement to care and attention.[5]

This is not easy. Fortunately, others have recognized this as well and have insights that can help us. In fact, research into institutional dementia care has yielded insights that can assist families as well.

From the Problem to the Person

The 1980s saw the beginning of a profound change in our thinking about dementia and dementia care: a change that began with some serious questions about the medical discourse I've described in the previous chapter, a discourse dominated by empirical investigation and the framing of dementia as a medical condition distinct from normal aging. Thomas Kitwood introduced a then-revolutionary approach to dementia care, by arguing that bio-medical research, while important, is not enough for understanding dementia and dementia care in a meaningful way.[6] No matter how carefully and rigorously medical scientists study dementia, they can't get to the full truth of the condition. Instead, Kitwood argued, we should think like poets and philosophers. When caring for people with dementia, we should stop measuring the severity of symptoms and instead teach ourselves to watch and listen. We should make what he called "a disciplined and thorough use of the imaginative and intuitive sensitivities that we use ... in trying to understand other people in everyday life." We should study the written accounts of persons with dementia; we should listen to them and observe them, both in individual and group interviews and in their everyday lives. We should consult those who've undergone dementia-like illnesses and engage in role-playing exercises to imagine how care practices feel to the one receiving them. We should risk abandoning our prosaic speech, which he deemed "too thin, too linear, too precise," and compose poetic, imaginative depictions of the dementia experience.[7]

What should we be listening and watching for, through our application of our imaginative and intuitive sensitivities? First, signs of retention: indications, however cryptic, that the loved one actually preserves memories and knowledge behind the impairments of speech, vocabulary recall, or short-term memory access. As we'll see in a later chapter, music can sometimes serve as a powerful mnemonic device: a person may allude to something familiar through a long-remembered song. Second, we should watch for indications of improvisation, as the loved one resorts to eccentric associations in words, signs, and gestures to navigate around the affected brain connections and express thoughts and feelings. Cathie Borrie's mother, as her dementia advanced, achieved a strange poetry as she struggled to express her thoughts: "I've reached the ultimate of the intimate and that's the end of it." Third, indications of response: signs that the loved one is responding to new and often unfamiliar predicaments, leading to reactions and responses that may, on first encounter, seem wildly out of character. Mary, for instance, was startled to get reports from her father's long-term care facility that her kindly father was lashing out at the staff. Inquiry led her to discover that these outbursts occurred when the staff woke him up in the mornings; further thought led her to remember that her mother had trained all the children from childhood not to disturb their kindly father in the morning. And finally, integrity: indications, however elusive, of a preserved character and an enduring identity, as Victor discovered when helping his father with his medications.

While Kitwood's approach may not bring us any closer to finding a cure for dementia, its widespread adoption has brought about significant changes in dementia care, particularly in institutionalized settings. Many care facilities, and the bodies that govern them, have adopted protocols that place explicit emphasis on empathy, respect, and attentive listening, particularly in stressful situations. The PIECES Framework for Responsive Behaviours, for instance, embeds empathy directly into its sequence of prescribed staff responses to behaviors such as screaming, biting, exit seeking, or wandering. The protocol guides the care worker methodically through a checklist that spans the spectrum of possible causes, beginning with physical and intellectual causes, but moving steadily through to possible causes rooted in emotions, changes in capability, responses to the environment, and possible social stresses.[8] As long-term care workers can attest, compassion need not be a spontaneous emotion: one can embed compassionate responses into procedures and protocols, thereby ensuring that staff exercise compassion, regardless of what they might be feeling in a stressful moment.

Kitwood's approach has given rise to a new trend in dementia care known as "person-centered care," exemplified by the work of Steven Sabat and his extended studies of persons living with dementia. Through repeated extended conversations with persons living with dementia, patiently attending to what they said and drawing on background information about their early lives and current circumstances, Sabat isolates numerous guidelines for clinicians and caregivers trying to understand the behavior and discourse of persons in their care. In one instance, he describes a conversation with a person who, when describing his frustration with using the telephone, repeatedly used the phrase "going into the yonder." With patient questioning and listening, Sabat discovered that the person was comparing his feelings about the telephone with his fear of flying, embodied in the phrase "going into the yonder":

> Clinicians must be relentless in uncovering background information regarding the dispositions and attitudes of brain-injured people lest they mistakenly attribute aspects of the person's present behavior to the effects of disease alone ... It is very important that family members and other caregivers be extremely attentive to the person's use of words, to look past the surface structure, and to use the context of the conversation as a guide in the process of "translating" what the afflicted person is trying to say.[9]

As with Victor and his father, Sabat was able to use background information regarding the person to distinguish behavior caused by the dementia from behavior that was in character; furthermore, he was able to use the reference to the "yonder" – an allusion to an American Air Force song – to follow the person's change of subject.

The person-centered care approach actively resists the imaginative framing of dementia in the context of horror and disgust: popular associations with zombie narratives of "living death" and other such pejorative and demeaning metaphors.[10] It aims to replace such terms with ones of empowerment, respect, and dignity. Above all, it aims to do justice to the full extent of preserved skill and enduring capacity and the resourcefulness of persons with dementia in improvising ways of expressing themselves and interacting with the world. We don't have to see dementia solely in terms of loss, of suffering, or of degradation. Our loved ones, with our help, can retain their capacity to think, to love, to laugh, to wonder, and to reach out to others for some considerable time past the point of diagnosis.

This is all very well. Except that such complex interaction is not easy. Here is Dr. Steven Sabat, indulging in some well-deserved pride over his successful interactions with a dementia patient:

> Throughout, I was providing him with a non-anxious partner in conversation, giving him room to speak, checking to see that I understood him correctly, letting him know that I wanted to understand and would work to do so. I believe that this approach was at least partly behind his comment, "Gee whiz, where is that guy? I need that guy!"[11]

Lack of anxiety. Time and willingness to listen, interpret, and respond. Compare this with Cathy Borrie's account of taking her mother to a doctor's appointment:

> Find handicap parking please God please God. Lift wheelchair out of the trunk open passenger door lift Mum out help her stand shift to wheelchair lift legs onto foot pedals oh careful push wheelchair up steep incline grind teeth against jabs in left hip go to appointment don't cry don't cry wheel back to car lift her out of the wheelchair into car clip seat belt kiss forehead lift wheelchair into trunk left hip left hip drive to mall for lunch lift wheelchair out of the trunk. In and out.[12]

Borrie's quandary is the quandary of all family caregivers. Family caregivers don't live stress-free lives. Empathic curiosity can be difficult when the left hip gives out while we're lifting a helpless person out of a car seat into a wheelchair. However much we'd like to see past the barriers to the human being we love, sometimes it's all we can do to deal with the logistics of the barriers.

Recent research on person-centered care has synthesized some findings that shed some light on this problem. In a thoughtful paper for the *Journal of Medicine and Philosophy*, two Australian researchers, Matthew Tieu and Steve Matthews, suggest that we in the West need to change the way we interpret the "person" who sits at the center of our care. Many government health policies place great stress on preserving independence, choice, and agency as long as possible: a stress that arises from a combination of consumer culture, from the influence of disability studies, and from a nervous desire to avoid massive public expenditure.[13] This leads, Tieu and Matthews argue, to an emphasis on what they call "personhood": celebrating the person with dementia as an independent and isolated identity, capable of "self-determination, self-management and consumer choice."[14] On the one hand, that sounds great: we should be consulting the choices and preferences of the people in our care; and in many cases, people *do* prefer to sustain their independence for as long as possible.

Except that independence is fragile at the best of times. Whatever illusions we may have of our own autonomy and self-agency get swept away when faced with age in general, and dementia in particular. The stories of carers are primarily narratives of recognizing that a figure on whom they once relied is surrendering to a growing and implacable dependence: of nearly setting a home on fire; of flooding a home and then disappearing onto the streets on a cold night; of losing control of taxes and finances; of setting out for a drive and getting lost. All this talk of an independent self feels incongruous when the caregiver is becoming increasingly wary of leaving the loved one alone.

Tiu and Matthews suggest an alternative concept, which they call "relational care." Relational care retains the core respect and compassion of person-centered care, but it grounds this care, not in "personhood," but in what they call "selfhood": a condition which is "essentially intersubjective, socially embedded, and depending on continuity of lived experience."[15] Relational care recognizes that we are all related to others and that our identities are intrinsically embedded in our social context. We are defined by our legal status, by our social status, by our economic status. And we are defined also by our friends, our acquaintances, our spouses, and our children. We make sense of ourselves through our interactions with this social context: strangely enough, we see ourselves better when we can see others, too, and can get a sense of where we fit and where we belong. Tieu and Matthews suggest that the task of caring for persons with dementia is not fostering some fallacious notion of "independence," but rather working to retain, as far as possible, their self-awareness:

> We think a better conception of PCC holds that the standing of an individual with dementia in care depends on a particularized acceptance within the social environment based on who a person is, where interpersonal interactions based on this can provide a stable platform for living, for continuing in some role, or more generally as a social agent.[16]

If we accept this notion of selfhood, the family caregiver's task becomes no less formidable, but somewhat more attainable. As dementia progresses, the family caregiver provides more than a sympathetic ear and more than the services of financial advisor and nurse and legal representative. The caregiver provides a vital connection to the loved one's sense of self, enabling them to recognize themselves within a shared communal structure. If we see Borrie's account of the wheelchair in that light, perhaps the most vital service that Borrie provided to her mother in that moment was the kiss on the forehead: a brief gesture that signified their bond in the midst of such stress and confusion.

Gestures such as these aren't always enough, however. Communication breakdown can easily rupture that sense of connection, driving the caregiver into frustration and the loved one into loneliness. We need tools to help us, and here is where communication research comes to our rescue.

Communication Research: Repairing What's Broken

In dementia care, the misunderstandings proliferate. Just about all forms of dementia sooner or later impede the person's communication skills, particularly as the condition progresses.[17] The vocabulary available to the person dwindles; distractions become more difficult to ignore; sophisticated nuances elude the person's grasp. As a result, conversations between caregivers and their loved ones suffer frequent communication breakdowns: instances in which one or the other conversant misunderstands or mishears the other. The collaborative act of curating an identity, as mentioned above, often flounders in the more irritating collaboration of simply trying to understand and be understood by people we've known for a long time.

For this reason, communication researchers have devoted considerable attention to a process they call "conversational repair":

> The series of events for conversational repair is collaborative, generally formulaic, and includes the problematic utterance(s), the signal of a problem and the repair of the problem. These events are collectively termed the trouble source-repair (TSR) sequence.[18]

Communication research has used the TSR model to identify useful strategies for performing this conversational repair, and these strategies have found their way into much of the practical advice offered by associations such as the Alzheimer Society of Canada, which advises caregivers to employ background knowledge, reduce distractions, use face-to-face interaction, be flexible in expectations, and use body language and tone to convey positive affect.[19] Nonetheless, communication breakdown persists and becomes more prevalent as the dementia progresses, constituting a significant source of caregiver stress.[20]

Effective conversational repair requires training and experience.[21] The caregiver must remain sensitive to signs that the partner has misunderstood or lost track of the conversation. The caregiver needs to be adept at identifying the trouble source, and ready with a variety of strategies for repairing it. Equally important, the caregiver must be sensitive to the loved one's own efforts at conversational repair, whether it be through voluntarily rephrasing, asking for clarification, or elaborating on the initial utterance.[22] While we naturally want to spare our loved ones embarrassment and stress, we can easily drift from compassion into officiousness, especially if our worry and exhaustion make us impatient.

As if that weren't enough, few particular situations remain constant over the course of the illness. If you're lucky, certain frequently repeated activities will endure for a long time, enabling you to work up a set of tactics. But as the disease progresses, communication strategies that worked for a time begin to fail. Changes might be gradual, or they might occur seemingly overnight; faced with such changes, the caregiver must improvise new ways of connecting, and find ways of interpreting new behaviors and patterns.

Finally, retaining communication as the dementia progresses involves more than simply interpreting ambiguous behavior to understand whether the loved one wants to visit the washroom or have another cup of coffee. As the cognitive effects of dementia increase, the questions get deeper, and more momentous, even as the loved one becomes less and less able to respond to them.

> What are your wishes, and have they changed since you last declared them?
> Do you have instructions about long-term care?
> Do you have end-of-life instructions?
> Do you feel safe?
> Are you happy?
> Am I doing it right?

These are tough questions, and most of us, even at full cognitive capacity, would be hard-pressed to answer them. In order to respond, the loved one needs a sense of self. Catriona Mackenzie calls this reflexivity:

> To be a self is to have a reflexive first-person perspective; it is to be able to conceive of oneself as a self, as having a subjective point of view that is distinct from other points of view and as the bearer of first-personal thoughts.[23]

The family caregiver is a vital link in the maintenance of that awareness: a vital witness to the fact that the person with dementia has a history, a family, and a place in the world. The family caregiver is someone distinct from the loved one, but who nonetheless belongs to the loved one. In the next chapter, we'll shift our attention from making ourselves understood, as caretakers, to understanding the enigmatic responses we receive from those in our care.

CHAPTER SIX

Categories

Communication researchers have given us useful advice on interaction in dementia situations. They advise us to use simple language and simple syntax when interacting with persons with dementia: not just because the simple words are easier to process, but because the person's sense of helplessness is exacerbated by a sense of incompetence and being patronized. They suggest adopting a moderate speech rate: slow speech taxes the listener's working memory, and fast speech creates information overload. They advise us to use choice or yes/no questions and to avoid excessive use of pronouns. They provide insights into "errorless training" and multisensory stimulation. Above all, they urge caregivers to capitalize on their own strengths while watching carefully to detect residual abilities in skills in their loved ones.[1] These techniques are invaluable when trying to make ourselves understood.

Nonetheless, when the loved one speaks to us, we may discover that "simple language" is not always that simple and that "error-free" interaction is a mere fantasy. After moving into assisted living, Victor's father telephoned him repeatedly, urging him to make sure the well in his back yard was securely covered. His tone was always calm and reasonable, but urgent: it took a moment for Victor to realize that the well was not at the home his father had recently left, but on the farm of his father's childhood. Ben's mother began encouraging him to date a woman in her neighborhood, forgetting what she had known for years: that Ben was gay. Jane's husband entertained visitors over tea with a succinct and detailed account of an incident from the week before. Only Jane knew that the incident had never happened.

As close family members, we cannot help but respond, not simply to our loved ones' words, but also their moods. We are used to listening to them with respect. And when they grow angry, frustrated, suspicious, frightened, or sad, we cannot help but pay attention. But how do we interpret the communicative gestures of our loved ones? What do we read into them?

Enigma #1: Implicature

In a 1975 essay, "Logic and Conversation," Paul Grice brought a philosopher's attention to a phenomenon intrinsic to our daily lives: conversation.[2] Making sense of all the diverse ways we humans all chat with each other would daunt most of us, but Grice produced four "Conversational Maxims": unspoken, unwritten but generally persistent rules that govern conversations between adult human beings. Elizabeth Ahlsén paraphrases these maxims as follows:

- **Quantity**: Make your contributions as informative as is required (for the current purposes of the exchange). Do not make your contributions more informative than is required.

- **Quality:** Do not say what you believe to be false. Do not say that for which you lack adequate evidence.
- **Relation:** Be relevant.
- **Manner:** Be perspicuous. Avoid obscurity of expression. Avoid ambiguity. Be brief (avoid unnecessary prolixity). Be orderly.[3]

These are very sensible maxims. Be informative; be truthful; be relevant; be succinct. Still, most of us are guilty of flouting them from time to time. We sometimes overshare with long-suffering friends. We sometimes spread unsubstantiated gossip. Anyone who has chaired a meeting knows the challenge of keeping the discussion focused on the matter at hand, and as an academic, I frequently stray into long grass and longer words.

Apart from these slips from grace, Grice argues that we also flout these maxims deliberately, for communicative effect: tactics which he terms "implicatures." When observing a tornado approaching, we might resort to understatement and say, "Well, this could be a bit of a problem." When suffering a minor inconvenience, we might resort to humorous exaggeration, and offer to chain ourselves to the office wall if someone doesn't descale the coffee maker. We use irony and sarcasm to belie the semantic content of our own words, relying on our listener to understand that, as Ahlsén puts it, "one can mean more than what one actually says." And this can become a problem when conversing with someone with a cognitive disorder suffering from reduced sensitivity to convention, context, the speaker's intentions, or semantic distinctions.[4]

Obviously, the caregiver needs to be aware that the loved one may not be able to follow the normal implicatures of conversation and may take something seriously that was meant ironically, or attribute exaggerated importance to a trivial event. But the problem goes deeper than that. In her famous story, "The Bear Came Over the Mountain," Alice Munro describes a woman with dementia getting lost:

> Fiona, who no longer went shopping alone, disappeared from the supermarket while Grant had his back turned. A policeman picked her up as she walked down the middle of the road, blocks away. He asked her name and she answered readily. Then he asked her the name of the prime minister of the country.
> "If you don't know that, young man, you really shouldn't be in such a responsible job."
> He laughed.[5]

In this scene, and indeed throughout the story, Fiona's responses could contain deliberate implicatures, and they keep others in constant doubt: how much of her speech means more than it says, and how much of it means less? Her response to her own lapses – "surprise and apologies [that seem] like routine courtesy, not quite concealing a private amusement"[6] – keep her husband, and the policeman, off balance.

In Cathie Borrie's account of her mother's dementia, her mother's responses keep Borrie off balance as well, partly because both remain haunted by the past, particularly the death of Borrie's brother at an early age. At various points, the mother confuses her daughter with her dead son: "you're the boy," she says once, "and you're my favorite."[7] It is unclear, to Borrie herself and to us as readers, exactly what the mother means. Has the mother simply mistaken the gender of the child she's addressing? Or is she implying that her daughter comes a distant second in her affections to the son she lost years ago?

What implicatures do we draw from the discourse of the loved one for whom we're caring? Do we try to find deeper meanings in the loved one's speech, in an effort to retain our sense of connection with someone with whom we once exchanged deep meanings as a matter of course? Or do we discount implicatures when we detect them in the loved one's speech – words and phrases that imply censure, irony, malice, or even surprising wisdom – and decide that it's just the illness talking? How responsible are they for what they say and what they imply? How carefully should we limit what we infer from the loved one's words and gestures and actions?

These are tough questions. If, as caregivers, we can understand more about how dementia affects the brain's ability to assign names to things and place them in categories, it may give us more resilience and flexibility when trying to make sense of what our loved one is saying or doing.

Enigma #2: Lost or Mislaid?

The brain has various memory systems, and the variety of names can be confusing. At the risk of drastic oversimplification, I prefer to divide them up into the following:

- *Procedural Memory*: the memory of how to do things, often called *implicit* memory as well. This is the memory that we use to perform automatic actions without conscious thought, and once acquired, we do them rapidly and automatically. We use this memory to walk, to drive, to perform regular daily tasks, to play a musical instrument.
- *Declarative Memory*: the memory of facts (*semantic memory*) and events (*episodic memory*). Declarative memory is frequently divided into long-term and short-term memory, and dementia can interfere with one or both. We use

declarative memory to recall names, both recently acquired and learned long ago, to know the difference between toothpaste and shampoo, and to remember where we put things and where we should put things.

Procedural memory can be surprisingly robust, which is why so many people with dementia preserve skills ranging from playing musical instruments to folding laundry. Declarative memory, however, is more vulnerable to change. How do we interpret the changes in our loved one's access to declarative facts, whether it be the names of the children, the phone number, the date, the name of the prime minister, or perhaps most importantly, precious episodic memories of a full and shared life? How do we interpret the surprising accuracy of some memories and the jarring inaccuracy of others?

Dementia research struggles with two contradictory hypotheses. One suggests that in cases of dementia, particularly dementia of the Alzheimer's type, the person suffers from gradual but permanent memory loss. The other hypothesis suggests that memories may persist, but that the brain's ability to access them has degraded in various possible ways.[8] This raises a vexed question for the caregiver: if the loved one no longer appears to remember things, is the knowledge lost forever? Or do the memories lurk in the brain the way a mis-shelved book languishes on a library shelf, waiting for some eureka moment when the brain manages to rewire its associations and find them again?

Whichever hypothesis ultimately predominates, the caregiver faces two challenges: that of helping the loved one to retain access to memories for as long as possible, and that of finding any patterns in the person's speech and recall that indicate how the memory system is changing as the condition progresses. These are questions in psychology, to be sure, and researchers in cognitive psychology are actively working on them. But on a more pragmatic level, these are also questions of knowledge organization. Library catalogues, databases, and search engines exist because there's more information out there than our minds can hold: we need tools that extend our access to information beyond our individual memories. If there's something important that we've forgotten, or something we never knew in the first place, we go to our tools – Siri, Alexa, Wikipedia, search engines, reference sources, friends, and colleagues – and get help. When we don't have the answers ourselves, we have to look them up.

If people with dementia merely needed to look more things up, and look them up more often, communication with the caregiver would be frustrating, but not especially complicated. We can label cupboards and drawers, so that our loved ones can find a coffee cup and a pair of socks. We can put simple passwords on a pad near the computer. We can organize their medication into pill boxes; we can help them find the vegetable section of the supermarket. Answering the same question over and over again for a forgetful parent or spouse can be tedious, but it's hardly a crisis, as long as the question is relevant and the answer appears to make sense.

Unfortunately, conversation with a person living with dementia can be rather more confusing. We're not merely dealing with the person's memory loss; we're also dealing with changes in the fundamental categories by which that person understands the world.

Enigma #3: Naïve Classification

There is a theory in psychology called "theory theory"[9]; in knowledge organization we have a related concept that we call "naïve classification."[10] According to this view, we all go through life with a naïve working understanding of how the world works. We know that the sun goes down at night and returns in the morning, that winters in Canada tend to be cold and summers warm. Within our daily lives, we put the vegetables in one crisper in the refrigerator and the fruit in the other, the dishes in one cupboard and the food in another; we expect to find a cash register at least somewhere in a retail establishment, and a "CONTACT US" button on most organizational websites. These naïve classifications may be misinformed – they may lead us to assume that all police are like the police in cop shows, or that the guy in a white lab coat on a Facebook ad really *is* a scientist, or that evil people in the world always scowl and wear black hats – but rarely do they interfere with the ordinary business of living. As George Eliot once put it, we all need times, particularly as children, when we can see the stars merely as friendly companions in our own backyards. There will be time enough to grasp the frightening scope of the universe later in our lives.[11]

Research in cognitive psychology, however, has discovered that dementia can change the basis of our "theory theories": those narratives we create that account for most of what we encounter in daily life. Much of our "normal" categorization tends to be in hierarchies. If you visit a public library that uses Dewey's Decimal Classification, you will find Canadian politics in Politics, music within Fine Arts, and dogs under Mammals, alongside wolves. If I go into a department store, I'll find ties in the Menswear section; if I want to buy a bed at Ikea, I have to find my way to the Bedroom section.

Thematic or "contiguous" associations, on the other hand, arise because certain things become associated through co-occurrence in time or place. And there is some evidence that persons with dementia gravitate from associations based on hierarchy to associations based on theme. In such cases, a dog is more meaningfully connected with a leash and a can of dog food than with a wolf or a mammal.[12] Then, as the condition progresses, even these thematic associations might drop away, leaving the person with only perceptual cues such as shape.[13] A carrot, for instance, may first be associated with vegetables; later, the carrot might be grouped thematically with rabbits, thanks to a lifetime of watching Bugs Bunny. Finally, the person might associate a carrot with something like a rocket, thanks to the long, slender shape they both share.

Here is where "selfhood," as mentioned in the last chapter, becomes important. As a person embedded in social and family relationships, the loved one's categories may well be determined by the specific and even eccentric nature of those relationships. As a family member with a close understanding of the person in your care, you may need to draw on memories of family life and family traditions to understand the connections the person makes between things which, to an outsider, make no sense at all. The connections may be thematic, rather than hierarchical, related to idiosyncrasies in the person's life that have remained more stable and meaningful than the hierarchies of the outside world.

Enigma #4: What Is "Simple"?

Naming patterns can create a further complication. While the guides tell us to use simple language, we find in some cases that simplicity and clarity are two distinct qualities.

Since the 1970s, research in cognitive psychology has accepted, to greater or lesser degrees, the existence of what Eleanor Rosch called the "base level of categorization." At this level, we name the things that are most fundamental to our environment, both physically and socially. When, as children, we first learn to speak, we learn at this level, and the words at the base level tend to be the most linguistically simple. We learn the words "cat" and "dog" at an early age, and as we mature we start to discover categories both above and below that level. We learn that some dogs are retrievers and some terriers; we learn that both dogs and cats are mammals, and that both are considered typical house pets, at least in some societies.[14]

Given the toll that dementia takes on cognition, we might expect that persons with dementia would retreat to an articulate form of "second childhood": retreating from the complex, poorly understood schemas of adulthood, taking refuge in naïve theories of the world, inhabited by entities that they describe in simple, basic language. That isn't always true.

Precision vs. Simplicity

When I teach library indexing, I'm always reminding my students: it's not enough to use simple words. We have to reach for words that are "coextensive": terms that are neither broader nor narrower than the subject of the book. If the book is about apples, index it with **Apples**, and not **Fruit** or **Granny Smith apples**. We need a term that not only places something in a category but distinguishes it from other members in the same category.

When the guides for dementia care tell us to use simple language, it's easy to assume that "simplicity" means base-level terms: terms that are old, simple, and direct, without burdening the person with hierarchical relationships that are often complex. Evidence suggests, however, that dementia patients do not always adhere to the base level.

For one thing, we are all subject to priming effects. When trying to remember facts or identify entities, we can be powerfully affected by the presence of a related stimulus. Think of Portia, in Shakespeare's *The Merchant of Venice*, helping her boyfriend choose a winning casket made of lead by playing a song in which every line rhymes with "lead." Patients with dementia sometimes exhibit an exaggerated form of this tendency called "hyperpriming," creating a greater tendency to false recognition and spurious categorization.[15] A mother with Alzheimer's, for instance, who has been pleasurably surprised by a rare visit from her out-of-town son might be hyper-primed into proudly introducing him as her primary caregiver, to the irritation of the daughter who's been slogging by her side for the last two years.

In addition to statements made in error, we also have the problem of statements that don't say much at all. As the dementia impedes their cognition, people are forced to improvise as best they can. And that sometimes involves retreating to a higher level which, if not defining the concept, at least includes it: in at least one study, "Patients were more accurate at verifying properties shared by many exemplars in a category (i.e. superordinate knowledge) than properties specific to few exemplars in the category (i.e. item-specific information)."[16] The language of the loved one, in such cases, exhibits simplicity without specificity, resulting in an increasing use of vague terms:

> When the attributes of concepts start being lost – whereas superordinate information is well preserved (e.g. the tiger and the lion are still known to be wild animals, but knowledge about their stripes and mane, respectively, is lost) – the ability to distinguish between two very similar concepts, such as tiger and lion, is impaired.[17]

Linguistic studies of authors Agatha Christie and Iris Murdoch show that the vocabulary in the words of both authors in later works became progressively less varied, with a reduced vocabulary and a greater reliance on vague terms, providing tentative evidence that Christie, like Murdoch, developed dementia in the 1960s.[18]

For the caregiver, then, interaction with the loved one, far from being the exchange of simple but pithy exchanges, might well degenerate into the frustration of trying to divine what the person means through a profusion of vague and near-meaningless words such as "thing," punctuated by specific references to the wrong person, the wrong place, or the wrong number, each of which, for some reason, stands out in the person's mind.

Conclusion

The "understanding mode," then, is a mode of listening, observation, and detective work. In contrast to the perspectives of our conventional, "real world" view of dementia, the understanding mode moderates the sense of doom and catastrophe that can easily accompany a medical diagnosis of dementia. The ability to communicate meaningfully with a loved one can last, if we're fortunate, longer than we might realize. Through the use of experimentation with different techniques, a willingness to change things up when existing strategies fail to serve, and careful and empathetic listening, we can preserve a rapport, even as it changes, for longer than we might have originally supposed.

But let's not pretend it's easy. More and more weight shifts to the caregiver as the condition progresses. Deteriorating powers of communication, coupled with decreasing predictability of association makes the empathy of person-centered care a matter of constant improvisation. And the caregiver becomes increasingly solitary in the act of association, retaining the signs and shapes of a former coherence – dressing the loved one in familiar clothes, playing old, familiar songs, preserving and recounting memories – that is becoming less and less real and relevant, as far as we can tell, to the person for whom we're caring.

With the loss of communication and the disruption of conventional, shared categories, the loved one becomes a mystery. And as the caring process continues, the caregiver emerges as a major protagonist. Far from being a passive companion who cooks the meals, pours tea, and performs basic nursing, the family caregiver emerges as the curator and prime decision force in the loved one's life: the one with the best chance of helping the loved one preserve a sense of selfhood.

And let's be clear here: preserving selfhood is not the same as preserving the past. The loved one is facing an entirely new set of changes: changes that are unavoidable and relentless. As these changes take their course, the loved one will change, too. The caregiver cannot preserve the loved one's past. The caregiver can only work to ensure that the changes remain consistent with the loved one's past, and that elusive voices from that past stabilize the person's sense of self in the midst of all the inner and outer upheaval.

That's a powerful and responsible position, and a potentially dangerous one. It forces us to look at the real world and our own internal worldviews in a new way. And that opens a fresh vein of questioning that requires us to shift from the "understanding" to the "advocating" mode.

PART FOUR

Taking a Stand

The Advocating Mode

Nobody is incapable of doing a foolish thing. Nobody is incapable of doing a wrong thing.
— Oscar Wilde, *An Ideal Husband*, Act 3

CHAPTER SEVEN

Facing Out

The nurses are working hard enough; you don't want to make it harder.
— Ben

I don't trust [the medical profession.] They're full of shit and they lie to you.
— Jeff

I think, as a caregiver, you've got to try to get fighting right. To fight only when, and for as long as, a particular fight serves a purpose. For as long as it holds out promise of helping the one you're fighting for.
— Mike Barnes, *Be With*[1]

Mike Barnes acquired his artistry in a tough school: the award-winning Canadian poet and novelist has grappled with mental illness throughout his life. What's more, he honors his condition as an ally in his craft, rather than as an obstacle to it:

> The experience of mental illness opens up windows and doors that, for a price, can show you a lot: alternative ways of being

and perceiving, the fragility of not only wellness but reality as constructed, the utility and costs of social conventions ... Going "away" mentally ... opens up your psychic pores – you develop finer antennae and broader sympathies for your fellow creatures.[2]

Mental illness, Barnes argues, has placed him at a distance, a critical distance, enabling him to stand outside the conventions and assumptions of a society that forms our understanding, not just of who is "healthy," but also what is "real."

Barnes put this painfully acquired insight to good use when, while caring for his mother in her dementia, he published *Be With: Letters to a Caregiver* in 2018. Taking the form of three letters addressed to a caregiver, he describes the caregiving experience in rich, diverse fragments of observation, using a poet's facility with metaphor and analogy to convey the wealth of emotions unearthed in the process.

Among these metaphors we find a metaphor of war and conflict. Dementia is a fight to survive: "There is such pathos and nobility in people's fight. Such a terrible dignity in the lengths they'll go to just to go on."[3] It is also a losing fight:

> A retreat under fire, I've often read, is the most difficult of military manoeuvres. You no longer hope to win, but bend all your efforts to forestall a rout; and you do so with dwindling resources and morale, foremost your own ... Dementia is retreat under fire. Caring for someone with dementia is retreat under fire.[4]

Both caregiver and loved one are "at war": always with dementia, but sometimes also with all of the institutional mechanisms and requirements, many of them well intentioned, that come with such a drastic loss of independence and self-agency. And as a caregiver, you frequently need to advocate on behalf of a loved one who can no longer assert the right for attention, care, and respect. Barnes acknowledges this obligation, but he frames it within a deeper obligation to "be with" the loved one:

> Arranging for medical attention, monitoring nutrition, hiring extra help, managing legal and financial affairs, talking to health care workers, buying clothes/drugs/toiletries/snacks, doing laundry – all these matter. A lot. All of the dozens of things you do for your loved one matter a lot. Being with matters more.[5]

This is what Frye called the "rhetoric" mode and which I call the "advocating" mode. Rhetoric is typically described as the power to persuade. Associated with the arts of oratory, it inspires us by appealing to more rapid responses than those triggered by reason and reflection. Rhetoric appeals to emotion; it invokes, not truth necessarily, but allegiance. Learning the truth of things is all very well, whether it be the scientific and medical truth of dementia or the elusive truth of the person living with it. But in the advocating mode, the caregiver needs to act: to secure what the loved one needs, to argue on the loved one's behalf, to manage what the loved one can no longer manage. And the caregiver does this, not because it's the "decent thing" to do for any fellow human being, but because of a deep, loving bond of loyalty and allegiance.

Furthermore, when acting as an advocate for a relative with dementia, the caregiver spends a lot of time scrutinizing other people's expressions of concern, trying to determine their source and their sincerity. Doctors, social workers, governments, administrators, neighbors, librarians, nurses, therapists, recreational directors: care and service providers of all stripes express a commitment to your loved one's safety and happiness. Often, we find the commitment to be genuine, surprisingly so. But limitations to that commitment appear in many different places, and as caregivers we must assess those limits as best we can.

Caregivers adopt the advocating mode frequently throughout the long experience of dementia care. But this mode is of the greatest importance at crucial junctures in the experience: particularly that juncture when the loved one needs to move into some form of assisted care. In so doing, the loved one is surrendering to the uncertain mercies of the health care system, and the caregiver's job is to ensure that those mercies will be as certain as they can be.[6]

Advocacy

In moving a family member into assisted care, the family caregiver must gather the choices that are available for assisted living, taking into account such factors as cost, the level of care required, location, and ease of access for visiting. Determining the range of choices frequently involves an analysis of the loved one's financial resources, and decisions as to how those resources are to be allocated; if the loved one is relentlessly determined to leave something behind after death, for instance, such a desire must be factored into the range of choices feasible.

The caregiver and the loved one together must evaluate the choices, taking into account medical assessments of current needs and prospects of future needs. The evaluation typically involves tours of facilities, checklists of features and services after which to inquire, harvested comments and feedback from websites and from any other information available, formal and informal.

Finally, the caregiver must ensure that the person, once established in the residence, continues to be looked after: watching for any signs of neglect or abuse, negotiating changes in care over time, maintaining communication with the medical and caregiving staff within the residence, visiting regularly and intervening in challenging or problematic situations.

All of these activities involve advocacy: actively and deliberately and openly working with various stakeholders in the social world, particularly in the world of health care, on behalf of someone who has limited agency. Advocacy has always been a part of dementia care – indeed, of elder care in general – from the very beginning, becoming more urgent in cases where the condition robs someone of speech or comprehension.

The Images of Assisted Care

When deciding that a loved one needs extra support for daily living, the choices can be confusing. Senior living in Canada comes essentially in two forms: for-profit centers for retirement living and not-for-profit long-term care facilities. Retirement homes require the resident or the family to support the entire monthly cost of living, while the costs of long-term care residence are partly supported by the government. Retirement residences are open, subject to availability, to anyone who can afford them; long-term care facilities are open to those who've been referred by a physician, although they typically have waiting lists.

The distinction is sometimes difficult to follow. Many retirement residences also offer graduated care options, in which the resident acquires greater levels of care when needed; they also allow the family to hire additional care workers to come in and assist with daily living. A retirement residence, therefore, may have dedicated dementia wings. Similarly, the same company that operates retirement homes may also operate long-term care facilities.

Whichever choice we make, we find ourselves looking at advertising, in the form of newspaper and magazine ads, TV commercials and especially websites. Canada's aging population has made big business out of products and services for the elderly, and companies like Extendicare, Revera, Atria (formerly Sienna Living), and Chartwell have populated their websites with alluring descriptions of life in their communities. Statements of care philosophy emphasize the dignity of age and the rights of the individual. Images abound of smiling residents living happily in community: engaging with other residents in leisure pursuits; playing host to visiting family members who share eagerly in the activities; embracing smiling staff members.

The messages emerging from these sites are directed at potential residents and their caregivers and declare the following commitments:

- To *comfort*: the photos show facilities that look prosperous, clean, and luxurious, similar to the photos of cruise ships and holiday resorts, and in all likelihood appearing more luxurious than the worn, lived-in surroundings of the prospective resident's current home;
- To *community*: the residents appear to be surrounded by far more amicable companions than the prospective resident currently enjoys;
- To *vigilant care*: the residents are tended to by trained care staff who are there around the clock to monitor their well-being, rather than enduring the well-meaning but untrained care of a harried and over-worked spouse or child;
- To *ongoing life*: unlike the biological model of dementia, the residence presents itself as the latest chapter in a life that still has joys and fulfilment ahead, and that frames old age, even in dementia cases, in a positive rather than negative light;

- To *the rights and the dignity of the individual*: that the underlying commitment is to the comfort and care of the residents.

These sites are carefully designed to suggest, both to caregiver and care recipient, that the facility offers more, not less, of what the resident needs – that the loved one will live in greater comfort, greater companionship, better care and further opportunities for an enriching life than would be possible in current circumstances.

The fact that these websites look like advertisements for cruise ships does not mean that they're lying. Nonetheless, support organizations like Alzheimer's societies very prudently offer checklists and decision guides, enabling the caregiver to ask important and specific questions when researching different homes.[7] Such checklists typically encourage the caregiver to ask three important questions. Is this a genuine and reliable care facility that meets the general standards of elder care? Does the facility itself offer the means for my loved one to enjoy a decent quality of life? Does it meet the specific needs of the person in my care, as well as my needs as the family caregiver? A checklist such as the one provided by the Alzheimer Society of Canada might include the following items:

- Overall standards and policies:
  - Evidence of accreditation and regular inspection;
  - Regularity of care planning meetings;
  - Policies regarding use of chemical and environmental restraints;
  - Availability of medical staff.

- The facility itself:
  - Cleanliness of facilities and attractiveness of the overall site;
  - Presence of good signage and safety devices;

- Access to other services such as dental care;
- Quality and appeal of food services;
- Meaningful recreational activities.

- Suitability for the specific circumstances:
  - Choice of private or shared room;
  - Convenience of location for visitors;
  - Facilitation of specific cultural and spiritual needs.

Specific checklists are very useful: touring a care facility, with or without the loved one present, can be an overwhelming experience, leaving the caregiver tongue-tied at those moments when the tour guide pauses to ask if there are any questions. But the concerns of the caregiver go deeper than what we find on those checklists. We may approve of the presence of grab rails in the hallway, and we may be reassured by the fact that the tour guide addresses every resident by name as we pass through the lounge. But moving someone you love who is cognitively and physically vulnerable into assisted living involves risks. There may well be unpleasant stories hidden behind those cheerful websites, and it's worth looking at them more closely.

Nightmare at the Corporate Level

In 2022, *The New Yorker* published a harrowing piece about for-profit assisted living facilities, particularly those purchased by private equity firms that have no experience in elder care. In such cases, the facility faces constant pressure to reduce costs by cutting staff and to increase revenue by adding beds, resulting in fewer staff caring for more patients. This in turn can lead to a higher number of falls, less frequent bathing, dehydration, malnutrition, pain, pressure ulcers, and infections. The data cited is stark: "when private-equity firms acquired nursing homes, deaths among residents increased by an average of ten per cent."[8] Similar research in Canada shows that "deaths from COVID at for-profit eldercare facilities far exceeded the rate normally expected in this age group, and far exceeded the rate of COVID deaths at non-profit and publicly owned eldercare facilities."[9]

When you dig into the "Who We Are" section of the website, you might find that many of the smiling faces at the top of the corporate ladder know a great deal about real estate, construction, acquisitions, joint ventures, energy, technology, and media. This is reassuring for shareholders, but a family caregiver will probably find greater reassurance if at least one of the smiling faces has experience in institutional eldercare and is capable of detecting and preventing elder abuse, as well as insider trading. To whom must all these experts ultimately answer? The residents and their families? Or the shareholders?

Now factor in all that we witnessed during the COVID pandemic: families watching helplessly while overwhelmed nursing homes turned to the Canadian military for assistance in providing the most basic nursing care. It's difficult to believe that the facility you're looking at on a website, complete with its photos of residents laughing with smiling staff in the midst of prosperous cleanliness, is telling the truth. When the doors close behind us, does the place turn into a chaos of neglect and misery?

Nightmare at the Bedside

As if these systemic issues weren't sufficiently frightening, we are also learning a good deal more about abuse at the individual level, particularly staff-to-resident abuse in institutional settings.[10] The World Health Organization defines elder abuse as "a single or repeated act, or lack of appropriate action, occurring within any relationship where there is an expectation of trust, which causes harm or distress to an older person."[11] The US Centers for Disease Control and Prevention has classified elder abuse into a frightening list of categories that includes the following:

- physical abuse, including inappropriate use of medications or physical restraints, and physical punishment;
- sexual abuse, including a long list of forced or unwanted instances of one body part touching another, or non-contact acts such as voyeurism or harassment of a verbal or behavioral nature;
- psychological abuse, including humiliation, disrespect, threats, harassment, and isolation;
- neglect, including failure to meet essential means of medical care, nutrition, hydration, and hygiene.[12]

One of my participants, Jeff, detected traces of homophobia in the treatment of his husband by the staff in his facility. Jeff went to the Ontario Ombudsman after he noticed marks of bruising, one bruise showing the imprint of a ring, and after a long process got his husband relocated to another facility. In 2018, a public inquiry revealed the details of eight murders in two different Ontario care homes by registered nurse Elizabeth Wettlaufer. When asked why Wettlaufer had continued working at one facility for seven years despite repeated complaints for medical errors and inappropriate behavior, the facility administrator confessed that the facility was chronically short-staffed and was always struggling to hire and retain nurses.[13]

So yes, sometimes the nightmare is real, and it makes for a powerful and frightening story: long-term care facilities, sold to us as little short of luxury resorts, that turn out to be factories of cruelty maintained to satisfy the dividends of shareholders. As caregivers, we can easily be haunted by such stories: how can we trust those smiling faces that promise to care for our loved ones? Are any of them truly on our side? And as the family caregiver, will I have to fight them all?

The Waking Challenges

For many families, the prospect is less dire but equally complex. Wickedness exists, to be sure, but as Bernard Shaw once observed, really bad people are as rare as really good ones. In many instances of long-term care, the level of care regresses towards a mean: sometimes great, sometimes terrible, but usually somewhere in the middle. The family caregiver has to advocate for the loved one in situations where allegiance, loyalty, and dedication are very difficult to assess.

To begin with the obvious: some people are better at their jobs than others, and as Oscar Wilde reminds us, the best of us are capable of making mistakes. Participant Ben was very pleased with his mother's nursing home but unhappy with the medical care, particularly when his mother fell, and the doctor missed the evidence of a fracture due to a mistake in the X-ray procedure. Angry as he was with the doctors, however, Ben spoke fondly of the nursing staff and the extra effort they put in to interact with his mother, to the point of occasionally spending their breaks talking with her in her room and engaging her in conversation. In a similar situation, George quickly acquired an ability to tell which of the nursing home staff were the best caregivers, and was vigilant for signs of neglect or aggressiveness: "When you're dealing with someone that has dementia ... you become their advocate ... So, I can be pretty nasty, but I – it's not that I enjoy being nasty, it was, like, I had to be nasty. Like, I knew when I had to put my foot down and say, 'This is unreal. This is ridiculous.'" Being an advocate for his mother did not mean taking on the entire caregiving team with unrelenting hostility. Rather, for George, as for many caregivers, being his mother's advocate involved vigilance and discriminating judgment, in order to identify when and where open resistance was needed.

If institutional caregivers possess their share of human foibles, so too do people with dementia. And family caregivers, who have lived with the person for many years, are only too aware of these foibles, many of which acquire greater visibility when the person is frightened, angry, depressed, or disinhibited. Participant Nancy's devotion to her friend, a fellow nun in a religious order, did not blind her to her friend's occasional tendency to see herself as "a kick above the common."

Sometimes, it goes beyond mere quirks of personality. Our loved ones are human beings, after all, and over the years, we've learned through experience that certain kinds of music, certain tones of voice, certain flavors of food, and certain physical gestures trigger bursts of temper. Over the decades, we acquire the skill of stepping around these land mines for the sake of peace in the household. We then watch with sick apprehension as institutional caregivers, who have many foible-ridden residents to serve, cheerfully step on those mines. Some people, like Ben's mother, don't like to be touched, even if it's friendly and even if it's necessary. Some people, like Mary's father, aren't very friendly when they wake up in the morning. Some, like Nancy's friend, cling to a sense of superiority, real or spurious. And in institutional settings where it is logistically impossible to accommodate every foible of everyone, clashes can result: clashes where the blame, as in most quarrels, is distributed among the parties involved.

Mary recounted her efforts to defuse a three-way clash between her father and his personal care worker, between the care worker and the staff at the nursing home, and between her father and the nursing home staff. "I'm a litigator," she said wearily. "I dealt with arguments for a living ... Some of the skills were transferrable ... But I found it really hard ... There was my own anger to deal with."

An added complication arises from the very mechanisms designed to keep assisted living safe and beneficial. In Canada, elder-care residences must report to governing bodies that measure their success as overall systems of service delivery, rather than their specific success in caring for any one person. In any assisted living facility of significant size, the logistics of managing all those lives are formidable, and group living inevitably requires a level of compromise and obedience. Meal times are typically fixed, and if only to spare residents with dementia the stress of choosing, the options are far less varied than one might expect in a dining hall that's been designed to look like a five-star resort. This can be difficult both for the resident and the relative: however much we may love equality as an abstract concept, it's easy to resent equal treatment when it inconveniences us personally. Most of us feel annoyed if we discover that a book we wish to borrow at the library has a waiting list of 350 people ahead of us, or if we have to wait twenty minutes for the next bus to come by.

High performance when seen from the sky is not necessarily a comfort on the ground: if your parent has suffered a debilitating fall in the hallway, it is difficult to be cheered by a report that incidence of falls has dropped by 35 per cent over the past year. But large-scale assisted living facilities have to measure their performance from the sky: to report overall statistics that hopefully measure the success of the overall care provision, but may not meet the specific needs of one resident. The commitment to the needs of the residents may be sincere, but it may be measured collectively, rather than individually.

This is not nightmare territory: we're not dealing with the massive betrayals of human rights I wrote of earlier. This is daylight territory: the tedious realm of human conflict that often occupies much of our adult lives, the whips and scorns of time that drove Hamlet into such despair. But how can we distinguish the daytime dreariness from the nightmare scenario? In acting as our loved one's advocate, when do we speak up? And when, on the other hand, do we simply groan inside and play parent, consigning loved one and care workers to separate corners until they're prepared to calm down and play well together? Everyone must decide that individually, of course. But as an information scholar, I'd like to suggest one further source of help: publicly available standards and best practices.

The Personal Care Level: Guidelines and Best Practices

Policy manuals make for dull reading. They're typically designed for us to refer to in a specific instance, rather than to read in sequence like a story. In print form, they're often in gigantic and unwieldy three-ring binders that get in people's way and fall off the shelves. In electronic form, they're frequently difficult to search and tiring to read.

Above all, policy manuals are intentionally devoid of emotion. There's nothing there to move us, to stir us, to inspire us. And therein lies one of their principal strengths: policy manuals tell us what we're supposed to do, no matter how we happen to be feeling. You could be brimming over with love for your fellow creatures; you could be heartily wishing them to the everlasting bonfire. It doesn't matter. You have instructions; you have a procedure. And if the procedure is a good one, at least some good will be done, even if the situation is stressful and unpleasant.

The other strength of policy manuals lies in their classification systems. It's a bit like lifeguard training: in addition to the other things they learn, lifeguard trainees are drilled in rapid assessment in an emergency: the kind of emergency, the distance from the pool's edge, and the appropriate assistive device to use to bring the person to safety. In the same way, policy manuals and best practice guidelines in dementia care map out the various challenges of dementia care, group them into categories, and provide instructions or suggestions for each.

Not all assisted living facilities may be willing to post or share their specific policy manuals, but there are best practices guidelines available on the Web which can help to frame your questions. The Alzheimer Society's 2011 guidelines, for instance, advocates a person-centered care approach to dementia care in assisted living centers, an approach founded on four concepts:

- honoring the dignity and respect of persons with dementia;
- sharing complete and unbiased information with persons with dementia and their families;
- encouraging participation of persons with dementia and their families in important decisions regarding care;
- fostering collaboration of persons with dementia and their families on an organizational level, consulting with them on issues such as policy, program development, and health care planning.[14]

The guidelines describe what person-centered care looks like at both the level of personal care and of overall governance of the facility, and it provides lists of things to look for in each of these four aspects of care. A familiarity with the facility's guidelines can be very helpful in distinguishing care from carelessness. Many of us, when seeking help, may have felt bewildered at the seemingly slow and laconic response we encounter. Some situations, however pressing they may be, require a careful and methodical approach that may look like indifference or reluctance. The PIECES Framework that I mentioned earlier contains precise requirements for documenting an incident of a behavior such as screaming, and a precise order of potential triggers to examine. The care worker, for instance, begins with a possible physical cause, then moves to intellectual triggers, then emotion, then capabilities, environmental and social triggers, each of which has its own list of possible causes.[15] A familiarity with systems like these can help the anxious family member to link the broader care objectives with the specific practices. Such a familiarity enables us to move past the smiling professions of infinite caring to discover how this caring manifests itself in actual practice. Some of the best care may in fact come from people who never smile.

Anyone who has spent time in assisted living facilities can attest to witnessing moments of deep courage and nobility on the part of some residents and awe-inspiring commitment and compassion in the staff. But staff have bad days as well as good ones. What's more, they sometimes have to do things that the residents may dislike: bathing, dressing, lifting, restricting movement, applying therapies that cause some initial pain. In cases of dementia, the level of care gets higher as the condition progresses, but also more peremptory, and at times more humiliating.

Let's be clear: the affect of the staff is an important factor in the choice of an assisted care facility. No one wants a loved one to be surrounded by scowls and bad temper all the time. Nonetheless, as caregivers, we cannot insist that all care workers in our loved one's institution be of uniform good cheer, nor can we guarantee that dementia care will not involve some pain, awkwardness, and suffering. The best we can do is determine whether the practices of the institution dictate reasonable and appropriate measures to take.

Conclusion

In this "retreat under fire" which is dementia care, then, who is on the side of you and your loved one? Well, if you've ever worked in retail, you know that you can't please everyone all the time. If you've ever worked in a library or some other organization that is committed to the general good, you know what it's like to be assailed by people who demand individual exceptions. And if you belong to a minority group – racial, ethnic, or gender, for instance – you know that many systems for the general good, however benign in intention, may contain systemic biases that bring unintentional harm.

When it comes to moving the loved one into assisted care, the caregiver must remain vigilant to the possible nightmare scenarios, while patiently (and wearily) dealing with the daytime ups and downs. Determining allegiance is a tricky business when dealing with institutions that are doing difficult work in trying conditions for a great and increasing number of people. The best the caregiver can do is to dig beneath both the smiling surfaces and the unavoidable sadness and poignancy, and determine, as far as possible, what the facility is actually doing.

If only that was where the work stopped. But once we start raising questions of loyalty and allegiance, it is difficult to keep our questions focused on the caregivers "out there." At times, those questions swing around to face us. In the next chapter, we will look at our own loyalty as caregivers.

CHAPTER EIGHT

Looking In

When I was thirteen, no older, my mother took to loaning me out, hiring me to be more exact, to anyone who needed help with a senile parent ... Joyless though my life was, I was still doing it six years later when my mother went the same way ... Nursing is not my chosen vocation, but just where I landed up.
– Alan Bennett, *Allelujah!*[1]

As we saw in the previous chapter, not all institutional care workers are responding to a higher calling to serve the elderly. While some do feel that way, others may resemble Sister Gilchrist in Alan Bennett's play. They just ended up there, in much the same way that family caregivers do: that's how the cards were dealt. For that reason, the laziness, bad temper, or reluctance we sometimes detect in institutional care is all the more upsetting: it resonates uncomfortably with our own moments of indolence, impatience, and resentment.

In the advocating mode, the caregiver learns to approach the various expressions of support coming from the health sector, the government, and even from friends and family, with a certain dose of healthy skepticism. Whether we're dealing with malevolent intentions hidden beneath smiles or simply with good intentions that could end up as mere paving stones to hell, we can't afford to take things at face value.

But caution and suspicion can be contagious, and they can spread into some very uncomfortable places. At times, caregivers find themselves the object of the very scrutiny they level at others. Sometimes, we sense it in the look of cautious scrutiny coming from the neighbors as the daughter stops by to check on her mother on her way home from work. Sometimes, it's not even cautious, as Mary discovered when she invited a man she was dating to a family brunch, only to have him take vehement exception to the way she and her siblings were interacting with her father. Sometimes, we find judgment lurking within a discussion with siblings who disagree with the caregiver's decisions. And sometimes, the scrutiny is inside the head: the voices that keep us awake at night, whispering in our ears. Have I done the right thing? Have I done enough? Am I getting this all wrong?

In this chapter, we'll look at how the test of loyalty and fealty that lies at the heart of the advocating mode can switch directions and subject caregivers to the same questions they ask of others.

The Single Caregiver

When a family member develops dementia, the rest of the family – spouse, children, close friends – must confer on how to assign the caregiving tasks. In an ideal scenario, the family members have different but complementary areas of expertise and willingly take on the areas of care that they can do best. Perhaps that's why old aristocratic families in England sent their younger children into the church, into law, and into medicine. Having a doctor to deal with the medical aspects of dementia, a lawyer to deal with the estate, and clergy to perform the funeral sounds like a great way to prepare for the future. Throw in a couple of nurses, a physiotherapist, an investment broker, and a bartender and the family has a lot of the important needs covered.

Not all families are as fortunate. And no matter how many wonderfully skilled family members there are, one of them tends to emerge as the primary caregiver. Author Paul Monette, describing the AIDS epidemic in the 1980s, speaks of a recurring pattern, whereby the person struck with the disease is accompanied first and foremost by a "buddy": "the mainstay friend and the one in the ring doing battle," while the rest of the family and friends form a protective circle around the two.[2] A similar pattern often occurs in family dementia care. It may be the spouse, who has the most intimate knowledge and the most "skin in the game," as participant Jane put it. Or it may be the child who lives nearest, as was the case with Heather Menzies, whose siblings lived at a greater distance from her and her mother. In some cases, the primary caregiver might be the family member with no children, as was the case with participant George, who took his mother in to live with him, sparing his sister who was raising children. And in some cases, such as Cathie Borrie's, there's simply no one else.

The stresses I'll be discussing are by no means limited to those who serve as the primary caregiver. They can be felt by all those who are intimately involved and even beyond: think of the caregiver's employer who has to cover the increasingly frequent absences of a valued employee and feels caught between sympathy and resentment, or the school-age child who resents a parent's time caring for a grandparent, and the ensuing exhaustion and ill-temper. However, the family member who serves as the primary caregiver experiences these stresses in the most concentrated form and with the greatest variety.

The Stresses of the Caregiver

Let's begin with the basic experience. The caregiver, whether living with the loved one or monitoring from a distance, is dealing with someone who is becoming more and more helpless, less and less able to communicate, more and more vulnerable to seeming personality changes and atypical behavior, less and less able to perform the basic activities of living. Let's imagine this experience, working with only a vague and uncertain diagnosis of the condition, and no clear indication of the duration, only that it will end in death, and that the process takes an average of eight to ten years.

But there are other stresses as well: stresses which tend to emerge at the point of a major change in the loved one's condition or of a major change in the nature of the loved one's care. The first diagnosis. A major setback, such as a stroke or a fall. The decision to move the loved one into assisted care. In addition to the intrinsic challenges of assessing the situation and evaluating options, caregivers can also feel under scrutiny: an uncomfortable feeling that our loyalty, our commitment, our priorities are being observed and analyzed and judged by others. The very scrutiny that one has been levelling at care centers and doctors and support workers and administrators and receptionists is now being levelled at the caregiver's own motives and priorities.

Scrutiny and judgment are oppressive enough when they merely comprise odd looks from neighbors over the backyard fence or tactful smiles from friends and colleagues. But sometimes the surveillance is happening within the family. And things get rough.

Family Conflict

The great cynic, William Shakespeare, shows us repeatedly how quickly families can fall prey to suspicion and jealousy. Most of us, one hopes, don't end up like Othello, strangling our spouses in reaction to malicious rumor. Nonetheless, when stress descends on a family, the dynamics of the family unit are put to the test. And research shows that family dementia care can sour family relationships and undermine family trust.

Sometimes, the stress may be simply logistical; when you have multiple people all trying to pull together, sometimes the oars get out of sequence. When Lydia's mother had a fall in the street, the police contacted the brother; later that evening, when the mother flooded her apartment, the superintendent contacted Lydia. It was some time before they were able to piece together the entire sequence of events of that stressful evening. If you're lucky, such events become anecdotes: harrowing at the time, but eventually things we can remember with laughter and a shake of the head. But sometimes, the pain of the experience lingers, particularly if it touches on deeper problems.

We can begin with a classic deeper problem: gender expectations. Yes, we've come a long, long way since the 1950s, when all the doctors on TV were stolid men and all the nurses were angelic women. And in dementia care, the age-old assumptions that women are inevitably expected to be the caregiver are eroding steadily.[3] Nonetheless, old patterns die hard, especially when the caring advances to the stage that requires significant nursing care. If you're the only daughter in a family, you may indeed feel like Sister Gilchrist as you perform all the duties of the sickroom, while your brothers hover outside, waiting for the moment when the crisis requires moving furniture or fetching the takeaway. And as Elaine Brody demonstrated decades earlier, female caregivers are caught between parents and children, expected to care for an earlier generation while bringing up a younger one.[4]

Women who are primary caregivers have reported various negative interactions, including disparaging comments from family members about the caregiver's competence, dissenting assessments of the loved one's condition and second-guessing the caregiver's decisions. At times, long-standing stresses in the family dynamic, either open or submerged, aggravate these interactions.[5] Cathie Borrie's care for her mother brought many submerged issues to the surface, including her lasting grief over her brother's death and her mixed feelings about her mother's remarriage. Heather Menzies encountered some skepticism among her family about her mother's condition, skepticism which arose at least partly from the her siblings' suspicion that she was raising the alarm out of psychological need:

> I was the emotional one, which by implication meant the weak one. Plus, my inclination to take care of Mum was suspect ... When I turned to Jan in Edmonton, pointing out how much Mum was slipping, how much I had to do for her ... she reminded me that "well, you do need to be needed." ... I imagine that's how she saw things, as a continuation of me taking on too much, whining a little because it wasn't duly noticed and appreciated. And I have to admit, that was me alright, at the start of this: still the eager-to-please little girl.[6]

Family discord can be deeply unpleasant, particularly at times of a significant crisis that requires a quick consensus and an immediate decision. In the anxiety and grief, family members can become suspicious of each other, questioning the motives of one and the judgment of another and the strength of another and the credentials of another. Why is John so urgent to get mother into assisted care? Where is all of Dad's money going? What happened to the andirons that used to be beside the fireplace?

Sanctity

This doesn't always happen, of course. There *are* families that get along and that make every effort to foresee and prevent such rifts and ruptures. Indeed, there are times when a caregiver receives loud and almost deafening praise.

As public and political awareness of dementia increases, family caregivers are coming into the spotlight as essential players in the years to come. Canada's Dementia Strategy acknowledges their key role, and Alzheimer societies offer multitudes of services that acknowledge what caregivers are experiencing and offer the means of alleviating the burden. Support groups. Respite care. Advice. Checklists. All these are helpful, but on top of that, we have increasingly formalized systems for expressing gratitude.

Caregiver awareness organizations such as the Caregiver Action Network, the US National Council on Aging (NCOA), and Share the Care are raising the profile of family caregivers through their promotion of November as National Family Caregivers Month, and in addition to the very real services they offer to support family caregivers, they also have a number of suggestions for how others can show their gratitude. The NCOA, for instance, provides a list of "Social Sharables": a series of images and suggested passages of text, seeded with hashtags, formatted for Facebook, Instagram, Twitter, and LinkedIn. Here, for instance, is a suggested passage for posting on Facebook:

> In continuation of #NationalFamilyCaregiversMonth, let's give credit where it's due. ♥

> For me, I'm celebrating #Caregiving because *INSERT YOUR PERSONAL STORY*.
> 💬 Tell me why you're celebrating caregiving in the comments. #NFCM #CaregivingAroundTheClock #FamilyCaregivers #CaregivingHappens[7]

These initiatives resemble many that took place during the COVID epidemic to celebrate the work of front-line caregivers. They speak to a need many of us feel: to acknowledge, in as public a way as possible, a sacrifice that threatens to go unseen and to assure exhausted and demoralized caregivers that their efforts are not overlooked. On a more modest level, the CareYAYA Health Alliance offers ways to show appreciation for family caregivers:

- Write them a card.
- Take them out for coffee.
- Compliment them.
- Help out with chores.
- Get them a gift.[8]

There's no question that family caregivers deserve praise. But they also need help. This admiration of caregivers by others at a distance, however sincerely meant, tends to characterize the caregiver as a saint. Balance this with the findings of a 2003 study of women caregivers. Their primary problems as caregivers included:

- Unfulfilled or missing offers of assistance;
- Unmet expectations for social interaction;
- Mismatched aid;
- Incompetence on the part of the potential helper.[9]

These are not needs that can be met with a card or a gift, with the occasional coffee invitation, or even with occasional help with the dishes. Borrie recounts a far more realistic intervention:

> An old friend calls.
> "How are things going, Cath?"
> "I can't do this anymore."
> "Yes, you can. You have to."
> "I need to lie down with a man but not a lover."
> "I'm opening the zinfandel."

Later, her friend says, "I couldn't do what you're doing, not for all these years." To which Borrie replies, "Neither could I."[10]

Caregivers are not saints, nor are they martyrs. Characterizing them as such can feel like a trap rather than a release: rather than work to reduce their burden, we simply cheer them on to keep doing what they're doing. We may be sincere when we say, "I couldn't do what you do," but in the caregiver's ears, it sounds a lot like "I haven't the smallest intention of doing what you're doing. Carry on."

A caregiver's capacity for endurance has its limits. There is always more to be done: always more that one could do. And when the caregiver's will gives way, it may not be the result of a major catastrophe, but a small problem that has happened before many times, and which now, for some reason, is no longer surmountable.

The Outer Limits

Where's the straw that breaks the camel's back? Research is giving us a more nuanced sense of caregiver stress, and numerous studies have isolated specific pressure points at which the caregiver is most vulnerable.

Perhaps most obvious is the problem of responsive behavior: in which the person with dementia is responding to some unknown stimulus through disruptive and sometimes upsetting behavior, such as shouting, biting, repeatedly asking for help, wandering, or exit seeking. As one participant in an Austrian study noted, disinhibited and frightened persons with dementia are capable of generating "an infinite number of swearwords, for which I would have got house arrest for two months if I had said them myself."[11] Behavior which violates our social codes can be exhausting, when it's not downright frightening. Even the most considerate and delightful houseguests can wear out their welcome after a while: living with someone who shouts and swears at you with no warning is not what most of us would choose.

A sense of incompetence can also be a pressure point, in two ways. Most obviously, caregivers can be driven to distraction by the sheer variety of things they have to do, from basic nursing to financial planning, and from home repair to dietary planning. Another factor, however, is a fear of interactional incompetence: a fear that our ignorance of a situation will cause us to act in an inappropriate way. This includes ignorance about caregiving: not knowing how to move someone, bathe someone, feed someone, and all those other things. But above all, it is a fear of being unable to communicate meaningfully, especially as the dynamics of communication become impaired by the person's growing confusion and memory loss.[12] This fear can afflict us all when we visit someone with dementia, and it can play a significant part in the tendency of friends and family to withdraw from close and regular contact. But it also afflicts primary caregivers as well, as the disease progresses and new challenges both to care and communication present themselves. The fear of "doing something wrong" can sometimes be paralyzing.

Another pressure point is isolation. Social situations become more and more challenging as the dementia progresses, and outings and rituals that used to occur with no apparent effort become labored and complex. Meeting acquaintances becomes fraught with anxiety; the ambient noise of restaurants and coffee shops disrupts the person's attention, as do the complexities of a menu and the many means of paying a bill. George's attempt to take his mother out to dinner foundered when she suddenly became angry with wait staff. On another occasion he had to explain to her two grandchildren when their grandmother suddenly became possessive and fought them over the right to hold a doll. "All my mom's friends left her," he reflected. "I'm still struggling with that to this day ... I found people were annoyed with the repetitiveness that dementia patients exhibit."

The caregiver, then, ends up sharing in some of the loved one's increasing social withdrawal. And as the tasks of care become more intense, the caregiver's capacity to enjoy social interaction diminishes as well. Respite care, which might be used to touch base with friends and colleagues and family end up as opportunities to catch up on sleep, do essential business that's been long delayed, or simply calm the nerves in silence. Cathie Borrie's description of going to dance classes describes the strange disconnect that can arise when a caregiver engages socially. The fellow dancers interpret her ferocious energy as simple enjoyment:

> Fun? Can't you hear me crying in the bathroom? My mother is ...
> I can barely get out of bed to come here, you stupid goddamn idiots!
> I would never say.
> "The Latin dances really suit you. You have so much energy."
> Shut up shut up shut up.[13]

So yes, the social isolation can be oppressive, as can the endurance of responsive behaviors and an ongoing sense of personal ineptitude. But there's one other, particularly rancorous source of stress, expressed most succinctly by one of the participants in the Austrian study:

"As a carer, you feel you have to care."[14]

Here is where the advocating mode swings around and bites off the head of the caregiver. Because the very question we ask of all those smiling faces in ads and at reception desks – "Do you REALLY care, or are you just playing the game?" – ends up staring you in the face. And the more people applaud you, clap you on the back and declare, "you are a *saint*, and no mistake," the more that question stares at you. Do you really care?

The Inner Limits

In George Eliot's nineteenth-century masterpiece, *Middlemarch*, the idealistic Dorothea Brooke marries a man she assumes to be a great intellect and great scholar and prepares to spend her life in glorious servitude to his mighty life project. In a very short time, however, Dorothea comes to realize that her husband's mind is lost in "anterooms and winding passages which [seem] to lead nowhither," and despite her best efforts, she is horrified to find her mind "continually sliding into inward fits of anger and repulsion, or else into forlorn weariness."[15] Many caregivers could empathize with Dorothea. Inner rebellion, restrained repeatedly and continually, is painful, especially if, like Dorothea, we have naively overestimated both a loved one's capacities and our own patience and endurance.

Why do we become caregivers? What spurs us on to take up that responsibility? In a recent study of family caregivers in

Singapore, three answers to that question emerged.[16] First, practical need. You're there, and you're needed. It's one thing that keeps society from collapsing all around us: we see someone in trouble, and we do what we can. We jump-start a stranger's car in the parking lot when the stranger's car battery has died; we call 911 and offer rudimentary first aid when we find someone injured by the side of the road. We lend a hand when a neighbor is moving something heavy or tools when the neighbor is doing a job of work. It's all part of being human.

On a more intimate note, we become dementia caregivers out of a sense of social obligation: it's what's expected of us. After all, this isn't some stranger by the side of the road. This is my husband. My wife. My mother. My father. Someone close to me, someone with a claim on my affection and my responsibilities. To deny my care, we think, would be "unnatural," like Goneril and Regan in *King Lear*, turning their father out of doors in a howling storm. This is the reason we would probably give most readily. He ain't heavy; he's my brother.

The third reason may seem less intuitive. We become caregivers for the sake of "personal value and fulfilment." In other words, we become caregivers because we actually enjoy it. On the one hand, it gratifies our sense of "filial piety" and accords with our acquired ethics of love and loyalty that are embedded into many religious teachings.[17] On the other hand, there actually *are* moments of intense enjoyment to be found in dementia caregiving, moments that are documented by other researchers as well.[18] We'll look more at those moments in the next two chapters.

In a way, these meliorating moments are part of the problem. If we were all inhuman monsters, we would feel no remorse at refusing to engage in care for our loved ones: probably because we'd have no loved ones, anyway. If all that motivated us were dreary forces of social and family obligation, we might do it, but we'd be a lot more vocal about demanding our rights and demanding better services. But what are we to do with those sparkles of genuine fulfilment, genuine laughter, genuine love that pervade an otherwise painful and tedious ordeal? This is where the guilt really takes hold of us: in a state of ambivalence.

Caregiving researchers define "ambivalence" as "the simultaneous experience of positive and negative feelings toward the care recipient."[19] Reaching a breaking point in an experience of unrelieved misery is tough enough. But reaching a breaking point in a state of ambivalence can be even worse. How can you reach the conclusion that you can no longer cope, when the mitigating factors are shining as brightly as ever?

Participant Jeff spoke of his husband with warm affection: of the times they shared, of the fun they had, of their many friends. When his husband developed dementia, Jeff became increasingly isolated, as friends dropped away over time. He remained with his husband, advocating fiercely for him, facing down doctors and care workers and administrators to insist that his husband get the best possible care. He dealt with his husband's financial mismanagement as the dementia took hold; he remained vigilant while the husband took to wandering at night out into the neighborhood; he cleaned up after his partner defecated on the carpet.

From my side of the microphone, Jeff looked like a hero. But in relating his experiences, Jeff could remember only his own anger and frustration: not just at the health care sector and the medical profession, but at his husband and, most poignantly, at himself. If he had to live the experience over again, he said, "I would have loved him more."

Conclusion

Even as caregivers scrutinize the rhetoric of the retirement homes that eagerly welcome their loved ones into assisted living, they grapple with their own motivations as they bring this move about. We scrutinize nursing homes and retirement homes for the slightest sign of cruelty or indifference: the smallest indication that the institution regards its inmates as the disposable remnants of an ageist society, as the less-than-human remains of once-useful people. But the research also suggests that many caregivers are no less worried about their own motivations, their own allegiances. Plagued by worry and stress that is framed as saintly endeavor, we wonder if we truly have done all that we can: was there nothing more we could do? Could we not have carried on further? Did we move her too soon?

This is a gloomy place to end a chapter, perhaps because the advocating mode is one which brings on the most lingering self-doubts, questions that persist long after the task is done, for better or for worse. In the advocating mode, we confront so many insoluble problems: not just with the loved one, but with the health care system, with our infrastructure of elder support, with the limitations of our families and the limitations of our own strength and resolve. In the next chapter, we move from the drearily expected to surprising flashes of the unexpected.

PART FIVE

Taking a Breath

The Imagining Mode

An aged man is but a paltry thing,
A tattered coat upon a stick, unless
Soul clap its hands and sing, and louder sing
For every tatter in its mortal dress.
— William Butler Yeats,
"Sailing to Byzantium"[1]

CHAPTER NINE

Creative Surges

Introduction

In the 1977 movie *The Turning Point*, Anne Bancroft plays a prima ballerina approaching the end of her career. In a pensive moment, she reflects on the occasional surprises that her aging body affords as she approaches retirement: "Even now, there are moments," she says, "when it comes together. The music, the dancing, the lights, the costumes."[2] Aging out of a precious life does not happen steadily: even as age and bodily weakness creep up on us, we are capable of sudden surges of strength and self-command. And this is particularly evident in areas of artistry such as music and dance. And it would seem in dementia.

Ballet dancers have famously short careers: the demands of their artistry require young bodies. In 2019, however, one ballerina experienced an unexpected career renaissance decades after her retirement. Marta Cinta, a ballet dancer in New York and Cuba during the 1960s, was living with dementia in an assisted care facility in Alicante, Spain, when she was selected as a participant in *Música para Despartar*, a program dedicated to promoting the therapeutic power of music.[3] She appeared in a video that has gone around the world, leaving very few dry eyes in its wake.

The video begins with Marta Cinta in her wheelchair, while a young man kneels beside her wielding a music device playing the opening of Tchaikovsky's *Swan Lake*. With a peremptory gesture worthy of a prima ballerina, Cinta signals him to raise the volume. She listens, poised for a moment, and then slumps back in her wheelchair, shaking her head slightly. The young man takes her hand and kisses it; at the same time, the music builds in urgency, and abruptly Cinta's eyes clear, and her arms rise. She begins to move her arms in time with the music, and many versions of the video splice in clips of a young ballerina dancing *Swan Lake*, highlighting the poignant accuracy with which Cinta replicates the original gestures of the choreography, and the even more poignant way she listens to the music, anticipating its shape and progress as it builds to a climax. And then, abruptly, her strength gives way; her arms fall, her head drops, and she sinks back into her chair once again.

Throughout the video, Cinta's face defies easy interpretation. She is clearly rapt in the music, and her face and gestures evince the grim focus of the artist. In her working life, after all, this music once demanded levels of concentration and physical exertion that most of us can barely imagine. Is she happy? Is it a delight to recall and relive this experience of a past life when she was acclaimed, applauded? Is it a delight to hear the music and feel the pulse of the dance once again? Or is it an agony to be reminded of her former days? Are her motions rejuvenating acts of joy or the remaining autonomic responses to demands on her body that she can no longer sustain? Is it kindness or cruelty to draw her out of her dementia-induced isolation to perform for the camera? And when the cameras are gone and the care workers have taken her back to her room, will she be better? Or worse? However we respond to these questions, there is little doubt that the video of Marta Cinta is deeply moving, as we watch her recover some sense of ownership over her past and her memories, as well as a sense of agency, as her body remembers moves and gestures and timings.

This fascination with the hidden stores of artistic expression that lie within people living with dementia touches on the fourth mode, which I call "imagining." For Northrop Frye, this is the mode in which we transform our experiences through our imaginations and in so doing reach levels of expression that impress and move others as well as ourselves. Beethoven witnessed the rise of Napoleon with the same mix of excitement and disillusionment that many of us feel when today's world leaders inspire us and then disappoint us. But Beethoven transformed that accessible experience into the Eroica symphony. Most of us fall in love at least once in our lives: Shakespeare captured what that feels like and turned it into *Romeo and Juliet*. For Canadians of my generation, Joni Mitchell and Gordon Lightfoot captured what we were feeling in our teens and twenties and transformed those feelings into art. Most of us have favorite artists whom we're prepared to swear were taking notes under our beds during long sleepless nights: they present our feelings back to us in the form of songs, poems, novels, ballets, and movies, transformed and preserved for us to take and possess. In Frye's terms, we attain an act of "possession" over our experience: we take something complex and multifaceted and use our imaginations to transform it into something we personally own, that we make part of ourselves. For a brief moment, Marta Cinta gained possession over her experience, through the remembered acts of dancing to the music of *Swan Lake*.

It's true: there are moments in dementia when the loved one's personality and awareness and engagement with the world surge into unexpected life. Sometimes, these episodes are deeply painful: witness George's experience, when his mother surfaced while he was performing the most intimate of nursing duties, causing them both to burst into tears at the son's sense of embarrassment and the mother's sense of humiliation. At other times, such resurgences can be eerily moving, in which memories and abilities rebound to an astonishing degree. Many such instances involve singing, dancing, or playing a musical instrument. At times, they appear miraculous.

This chapter shifts the view, however, to that of the caregiver: the young man who kissed Marta Cinta's hand, the caregivers who washed and dressed her before she appeared and who took care of her after the cameras had gone. What is the role and responsibility of the caregiver in such instances? And what can the caregiver infer from witnessing a formerly mute and listless loved one suddenly rising into awareness at the sound of a familiar tune?

The Miracle of Art

The shift in recent decades towards person-centered care has been beneficial for researchers as well as for care recipients. When the person you care for ceases to be socially defined exclusively as a logistical problem and a drain on resources, it creates conceptual room for us to see the person's remaining and persistent strengths in addition to the growing vulnerability that so often preoccupies us. And as we turn our attention to the legitimate claims of persons with dementia to dignity and respect, the attention of researchers ceases to be focused solely on the melancholy measurement of "what was" and becomes free to explore "what is." What is going on in the minds of the people we're caring for, and how do the remnants of their former lives persist in transformed and sometimes beautiful current manifestations?

Hints began to appear in the medical and nursing literature in the 1990s, bringing some tentative empirical verification that while much is taken in dementia, certain things abide. In 1999, a team of researchers published a longitudinal study of a single person with dementia, who had been a piano player through most of her life. Over three years of progressive cognitive decline, the woman exhibited measurable deterioration in her ability to recognize songs, to transpose from major to minor keys, and to grasp other principles of music, such as meter and rhythm. However, her motor skills, when playing familiar songs, remained largely intact, with only minute and subtle losses in musicality; she was also able to transfer her skills from the piano to the xylophone.[4] In another study, a violinist with moderate Alzheimer's disease was able to learn a new song published since the onset of his dementia, showing an ability to retain musical memory far better than his memory for words, figures, or environmental sounds.[5] Oliver Sacks, in *Musicophilia: Tales of Music and the Brain*, wrote of incidents even more eerie and striking: of an opera singer, for instance, who had to be helped to dress himself and to be led onstage, but who, once onstage, performed an aria brilliantly.[6] The popular press has noted that singer Tony Bennett continued to be musically active, despite having Alzheimer's disease.[7]

A particularly vivid depiction of the power of music came in 2011 with the release of the film *Alive Inside*. In this documentary, Michael Rossato-Bennett introduced us all to a project in which persons with dementia were given iPod playlists composed of music from their various pasts. The film provides startling and moving evidence of persons' memories leaping to life at the sound of familiar music. In the most widely circulated clip, a man named Henry stirs out of his inertia at the sound of his favorite music on an iPod. The music inspires him not just to listen, and not just to sing along, but to speak, movingly, of the significance of Cab Calloway's music:

> It gives me the feeling of love, romance. I figure right now the world needs to come into music, singing. You've got beautiful music. Beautiful, lovely. And I feel the band of love, of dreams. The Lord came to me and made me holy. I'm a holy man. So he gave me these sounds.[8]

Bolstered by such astonishing evidence, many associations and care facilities have launched programs that seek to tap this imaginative "lode" in the lives of persons with dementia. Anne Davis Basting has developed a "creative care" approach that involves using theatre and improvisation to enable elderly persons, particularly those living with dementia, to get in touch with their imaginations and creativity: "Our vision was to bring together university arts students and professional artists together with a long-term care community to collaboratively create a work of art that could transform the community into a place of storytelling and meaning-making."[9] Various projects have flourished using art, dance, and music therapies to improve the quality of life for those living with dementia. And many Alzheimer societies, together with their local communities, engage in intergenerational projects such as choirs, enabling persons with dementia, their caregivers, and members of the community to sing together. Such projects provide moving evidence of pleasure and joy, involving pride of achievement, as well as stimulation and positive interaction with persons of different ages and at different walks of life.

Many of these examples look like magic: powerful evidence of what remains for persons with dementia, even after they have lost many basic life skills. They form an important counterbalance to the prevailing assumptions that dementia is defined solely by helplessness and emptiness. Oliver Sacks, appearing as a commentator in *Alive Inside*, comments on Henry's response to the music:

> The philosopher Kant once called music the "quickening art" and Henry is being "quickened." He's being brought to life … The effect of this doesn't stop, because when the headphones are taken off, Henry, normally mute and virtually unable to answer the simplest yes or no questions, is quite voluble … So in some sense, Henry is restored to himself. He has remembered who he is and he's reacquired his identity for awhile through the power of music.

Imagine how this prospect might move and inspire family caregivers. Loved ones who have withdrawn into passivity and indifference suddenly re-emerge into something like their former selves, with memories, feelings, words, and imagination. Suddenly, they are thoughtful once again, curious once again, able to feel and express love once again. Imagine getting a beloved companion back once again, making you realize afresh just how sorely you've missed the connection, the intimacy, the sharing.

And now, let's look at two small details in Sacks's commentary. First, the good news: the effect "doesn't stop." After the earphones are removed, the effect of the music lingers. But then comes the bad news: the effect lingers only "for awhile." Henry is restored to himself "for awhile." The loved one has returned, for awhile. Only for awhile. Music therapy may be a wonderful thing for persons with dementia. But we need to consider the impact on the caregiver of witnessing the ensuing surge and ebb of awareness.

The role of stress in dementia caregiving sometimes overwhelms our awareness of the role of grief in caregiving. There is much to worry about when caring for a loved one with dementia, but there is also much to mourn. A 2010 survey of research into caregiver grief makes two important points. First, the grief that we experience before the loved one dies is comparable to the grief we experience afterwards; it is no less powerful and no less implacable. Second, a significant factor in caregiver grief relates to what researchers call "ambiguous loss." This is the suffering we feel, not through the steady loss of the loved one's faculties, but through the unpredictable ways in which the loved one's faculties appear to fade and then return and then fade again:

> In ambiguous loss, the intermittent nature of the phenomenon sets up a mixed set of expectations that creates a revolving door of hope followed by disappointment and then ending in despair and a sense of being trapped and helpless by one's own situation.[10]

Seeming miracles such as Henry's burst of awareness in *Alive Inside* are impressive, but they can also be a double-edged sword from the caregiver's perspective, offering genuine joy but also genuine grief when the stimulation of the music wears off. To spare caregivers unfounded hopes and the ensuing sadness, we should pay closer attention to the research into programs that make extensive use imaginative stimuli, in the form of music, art, and dance.

The Evidence

Let's begin by looking at the evidence: what do projects such as music and art therapy actually achieve? And at the very outset, we must make an important distinction. Participatory arts programs are not the same as music or dance programs offered in institutional care settings, either through recreational programming or through therapy programs that involve activities such as art. Recreational programs are designed to provide enjoyment and to enhance the quality of life of institutional residents. They can vary widely in quality, depending on the institution's resources and the talent available, but they serve primarily to improve morale, enhance social interaction, and provide physical and mental stimulation to the residents. Art therapy programs exist not to enhance artistic ability but to alleviate specific symptoms.[11]

Participatory arts programs also seek to improve the quality of life for persons with dementia, but they are more ambitious. They generally involve the participation of a skilled artist, such as a musician or painter or dancer, and they seek to inspire persons with dementia to aspire, to learn, and to grow. Such programs, to be sure, seek to improve the mood, enhance one's relationships, reduce isolation, and provide sensory stimulation.[12] But participatory arts programs are founded on a conviction that such benefits can accrue most powerfully through learning, discipline, and the acquisition of new skills. Most provocatively, such programs are founded on the conviction that many persons with dementia are capable of aspiration and ambition: that not only can they remember how to do old things, but they can learn how to do new things, through the influence of dancing, painting, singing, acting, directing, and writing.

Do such projects work? It depends on what you're hoping for. Systematic reviews of such therapies carried out by the Cochrane Library are noncommittal, perhaps because many empirical studies seek to measure the effects of such therapies solely on the measurable facets of persons with dementia, and particularly their cognition: "the neuroscientific approach tends to examine music as an isolated phenomenon ... and to examine it solely in terms of its ability to effect change."[13] A review of dance therapy research found no evidence of benefit,[14] while the results of art therapy studies were inconclusive.[15] Evidence for music therapies is also inconclusive,[16] partly because such therapies are very difficult to measure and assess.[17] One study suggests that music therapies provide some relief of depression and anxiety but found no evidence of beneficial effects on cognition or on agitated or aggressive behavior. Other research is more optimistic, but cautiously so, and insists that we need better models of evaluation and better clinical trials to be more certain.[18]

Do these efforts to stimulate connection through creativity and imagination, then, serve any purpose? If we're looking for miracles, no. Empirical research characteristically rains on the parade of miracle cures, and even the inspiring examples of Henry in *Alive Inside* and Marta Cinta in that viral YouTube video don't pretend that the effect is lasting. That does not mean, however, that such therapies and activities are useless. If we shift our expectations to reality rather than to miracles – that is, if we focus on alleviation rather than on restoration – the answer begins to look very different.

To begin with, no one seems in any doubt: music makes for a good time. Nursing and retirement homes have been hosting sing-along sessions for decades, knowing through experience that such sessions are popular and good for resident morale. Studies of the more deliberate music therapy programs that have recently appeared, including iPod playlist programs, have shown that whatever these programs do or fail to do for the cognition, they have a beneficial effect on emotional well-being.[19] And increasing the happiness of a loved one, even for a little while, is certainly worth considering.

Another important clue lies in a study of training formal caregivers in assisted living facilities in music interventions. The study concluded, "Training for staff in live music interventions may benefit the delivery of person-centered care by supporting communication, easing care, and capacitating caregivers to meet the needs of persons with dementia."[20] The analysis suggests that the recipients of benefit were not confined to the patients but extended to the staff: the music intervention training enabled them to perform person-centered care more effectively. In other words, programs such as music therapy may have a galvanizing impact on the caregiver as well as the care recipient, and it would be worth looking more closely at that impact.

Caregivers, both personal and institutional, occupy an ambiguous position in projects such as the iPod initiative that inspired *Alive Inside*, or the study that brought Marta Cinta to the world one last time. At times, they seem invisible: figures like Martha in the Christian Gospels, who misses out on all the sermons and miracles because she's in the kitchen preparing lunch. Caregivers are the ones who make sure residents are in the music room when the musician arrives; caregivers are the ones who deal with the exhausted loved one afterwards and perform all the unglamorous tasks while the rest of us are applauding the miracle of song.

At other times, caregivers appear as catalysts. Like the young man who kisses Marta Cinta's hand when she appears reluctant, they serve as trusted figures. In a world that has grown too confusing to deal with most of the time, their encouragement inspires the loved one to turn the attention outward and engage once more with others. And in addition to encouragement, caregivers provide presence and witness. Yvonne Russell, the recreation director of Henry's facility in *Alive Inside* gently monitors Henry's experience, helping with the headphones and watching him. Later, she breaks into tears as she describes how it feels to observe the residents reacting to music.

Russell's presence, and her emotional involvement, may well signify the most important aspect of the iPod experiment. Another experiment suggests a possible reason why. In a study reported in 2014, researchers conducted a series of weekly music therapy sessions with 16 dementia patients in a Spanish nursing home, expecting that the sessions would improve their morale and their interactions with each other. No one was surprised to discover that the patients' emotional state improved. But the researchers were surprised to find that the patients' communication with each other decreased. Surely, they thought, that was wrong. Surely the residents would engage *more* with their environment and not less.

The researchers advanced a suggestive hypothesis to account for this counter-intuitive finding. In the surprised stimulation provided by the music, the residents looked with greater intensity to the music therapist conducting the session, rather than to each other. If their hypothesis is true, the persons with dementia did not awake to join a party but to connect intensely with a nearby guide.

Conclusion

What can we draw from this? First, surges of awareness do happen, often but not always in the context of some aesthetic stimulation which brings out some creativity, however rudimentary. Furthermore, programs that foster imaginative creativity such as singing, art, and dance have a beneficial effect on the lives of our loved ones.

Second, such stimulation requires presence and witness. Participatory arts programs are not merely something to keep people amused so that the caregiver can do other things. Instead, such programs are instead platforms for intense connection. As researchers in Norway discovered in their study of theatre projects for persons with dementia, participatory arts programs can trigger intense recognition: not just for the actors, but for the audience as well. And that can be frightening. Anne Davis Basting, in the study which formed the basis of her creative care program, implicitly brings caregivers into the equation by deliberately tackling the societal inhibitions that prevent caregivers from fully participating in the lives of their loved ones: "This book emerges from a single basic question: to what extent do our fears about dementia and aging contribute to the tragic conditions of living with dementia and the catastrophic economic story of dementia?"[21]

This is a disturbing question. What exactly *are* we afraid of when caring for someone with dementia? Tapping into creativity and imagination, it seems, has much to do with the caregiver: it gives a profound shape to the caregiver's fears and the caregiver's sadness. This willingness on the part of the caregiver to bear witness and be moved, to be open to a fresh and unexpected connection with the loved one even at the cost of some pain, comprises the core of the imaginative mode.

In the next chapter, then, we will shift our attention partly away from the imagination of the loved one to embrace the imagination, the creativity of the caregiver. The imaginative mode is a mode that intimately involves both. And while the connection need not be a musical one – not everyone likes singing songs, after all – I will be using some of the fundamental principles of music as a means of demonstrating what this mode can look like.

CHAPTER TEN

Pleasure

> Come down, O maid, from yonder mountain height.
> ...
> For Love is of the valley.
> – Tennyson, *The Princess*, Part 7, 178, 184[1]

So wrote Tennyson in 1847, calling down all those people who climb mountains to get a glimpse of the divine. In the previous chapter, I threw some cold water on the popular notion of music as a "miracle mountaintop" for people with dementia. I argued that while creative therapies such as music and dance and art programs have great potential value, they must be designed "in a valley": developed upon realistic principles of melioration and alleviation. Also, the caregiver must be involved as a participant, willing to be touched and changed by an experience which is often profound, if not always joyful.

But how should a caregiver be involved? Not all of us play musical instruments. And while I suppose every human creature has a song to sing, not all of us are like Florence Foster Jenkins, eager to share our problematic talents with the world. What's more, music therapy programs may not be available; or if they are, the task of involving the loved one in them may be prohibitively difficult. After you've driven someone with dementia to an inter-generational choir rehearsal and then back home again, you may be too exhausted to dance as if no one is watching.

The good news: activities that involve the creative arts do not provide the only way in which the caregiver can function in the imaginative mode, as I'm defining it. There are many other ways which caregivers have discovered by trial and error. In order to understand them, we need to get beyond the specific realms of music, dance, and art. We need to figure out how imaginative connection can take place anywhere. To do that, ironically, we have to move in closer to at least one of these arts, to isolate and identify the characteristics that stimulate imaginative awareness, not just in the loved one but in the caregiver as well.

In this chapter, therefore, I'd like to return to the subject of music, but not from the perspective of music therapy or participative arts. Instead, I want to look at music itself: how it is produced and our psychological theories of how music affects human beings. My goal is to extract principles and features that enable the creation of moments of intimate connection between the caregiver and the loved one: moments that are imaginative, transitory, and mutually created and sustained. Such moments are rare at the best of times and transient at all times. They remain, however, deeply precious.

How Is Music Made?

What can we learn about music as a means of connection between the loved one and the caregiver? If we start with the basic physics, music is a sound: a vibration in the air and upon the eardrum. More specifically, it is sound in the form of a sine wave: a vibration sustained at a specific frequency of oscillation between expansion and compression, frequently attained by creating the vibration between two stable points. The pitch of the sound is determined by the frequency: the rate at which the crests and troughs of the oscillation take place over time. The "loudness" of the sound is determined by the amplitude: the degree of displacement from resting position.[2]

Music has, then, four qualities:

- **Connection**: between the source and the recipient;
- **Stability**: the connection holds at a steady frequency;
- **Pitch**: produced by the speed of vibration;
- **Volume**: produced by the amplitude of the vibration.

Now let's look at a moment of connection between Cathie Borrie and her mother.

> My mother and I sit side by side on her couch and watch the November wind strip leaves off the trees. We watch the sea as the days grow darker. Shorter.
> "I wouldn't be alive it if wasn't for you."
> "Don't remind me, Mum!"
> "Aren't we amusing today."
> "Tell me about the sky."
> "Oh, I don't know about the sky. It's pretty beautiful ... but you have to wear gloves because it puts fingerprints on it and you don't want that."[3]

The two are alone, sitting quietly, and isolated from distractions. They connect in a conversation, each speaking directly to the other. The mood is calm: neither appears agitated or anxious. The mother appears to have no trouble recognizing the playful implicature of "Don't remind me," and responding with an ironic reply: "Aren't we amusing today." What's more, they both appear idly interested in the view outside the window, looking at the sky. The tone is gentle and unforced, idle but engaged. But what are we to make of the mother's talk of fingerprints on the sky? You can't touch the sky; her comment makes no sense. And yet, in a way, it does, and music provides a helpful analogy for recognizing that elusive sense.

Harmonics

In music, the tone produced by the vibration, particularly the vibration of a string or a reed, contains various components known as "harmonics" or "overtones." These harmonics occur at an integer multiple of the base frequency.[4] If, for instance, a string is vibrating at a frequency of 440 beats per minute, the second harmonic vibrates at twice the frequency (880 beats per minute). And if you lightly touch the string at exactly the halfway point, the harmonic rings out: the same note, but an octave higher. If you touch the string at exactly one third or two thirds of the string, you will hear the third harmonic, vibrating at three times the base frequency (1,320 beats per minute), a fifth higher still from the second harmonic. The notes produced by these harmonics are different from the original note played at base frequency. They are, however, "nested" within that original note. They don't disrupt or interfere with the original note; they align with it, giving the note added resonance and brightness.

The concept of harmonics presents a useful insight into the caregiving experience by offering a way to imagine multiple levels of connection and recognition that sustain our morale in the face of the loved one's failing memory. In connecting with a person with dementia, we can often find that our interaction is taking place on two different levels of understanding. Sometimes, that creates a painful discordance: irrational hostility and suspicion, agitation or depression, and sometimes utter incomprehension. Mike Barnes describes his mother's failure to comprehend technological devices such as the television and telephone and shower controls, as well as the arguments they had, with his mother's "wild, glaring eyes, a panic in her face, tears sometimes," and the "nagging cycles of call and response that circled a grievance perseveringly."[5] In such cases, personality change, or depression and aggression fueled by panic and bewilderment, create an implacable rift, at least for the time being.

At times, however, the two levels of interaction are curiously consistent with each other. Alice Munro, in "The Bear Came Over the Mountain," captures the ambiguous nature of Fiona's interaction with her husband when he visits her in the nursing home, and he cannot tell if she recognizes him: "He could not decide. She could have been playing a joke. It would not be unlike her. She had given herself away by that little pretense at the end, talking to him as if she thought perhaps he was a new resident."[6] Fiona's behavior is confusing, but it is strangely in character, as if both she and her husband are singing at different pitches, but pitches that are consistent with each other.

Sometimes, the caregiver is able to recognize the remnants of patterns from the loved one's earlier life and use them to make sense of seemingly baffling behavior. Tina's mother was once the manager of a senior's home; Tina found that her mother's criticism of her home care and then her assisted living conditions made more sense when she remembered her mother's former job and superimposed that upon her current behavior.

Other times, the parent/child relationship can survive a reversal of roles: Lydia found that her mother's behavior made the most sense if she compared her to a toddler. Similarly, Victor, who had spent his childhood holding tools for his father, now found a new tranquility in the later stages of his father's illness through the assembly of toy robot dinosaurs; he would construct the robot, with his father holding the pieces of metal and balsa wood and handing them over when needed. Indeed, George sustained himself in performing basic nursing tasks by framing it as a harmonious role reversal: "I took the attitude that, you know, she changed my diapers when I was a baby; it's time to just suck it up and do it. And I did it."

In many of the interchanges between Cathie Borrie and her mother, then, the mother's responses make little overt sense. They do, however, capture the quality of interchanges in which the meaning levels of the two conversants, while different, are somehow harmonious. The effect is whimsical, rather than jarring. Nonetheless, there is more, I think, in Borrie's conversations with her mother than the tranquility of two parallel lines that never collide. Some kind of connection is taking place. Can we get any closer to it?

What Does Music Mean?

What, then, are the caregiver and the loved one exchanging in the imagining mode? Let's go back to music, and this time ask, not how music is physically produced, but how it conveys meaning. What is the music telling us? According to Henry from *Alive Inside*, the music that he's listening to is about love, and it's a message that the world urgently needs to hear. How does that happen? Some music has words, certainly; music also connects to past memories. But music itself is a curious phenomenon, one that Stephen Sondheim characterized as "the richest form of art. It's also abstract and does very strange things to your emotions."[7] How does someone like Henry derive the sense of love from Cab Calloway's music? Is it a message? And if so, is it a deliberate message from the composer to the listener?

Music theorists tend to agree that music has the power to refer to things outside itself. Even without lyrics, Vaughan Williams can evoke the sounds of London street-sellers in his second symphony, and Tchaikovsky can celebrate battles in his *1812 Overture*. But music is not like language; it doesn't "tell us" things the way words do. Vivaldi's *Four Seasons* contains sounds that bear some resemblance to the sounds of birds singing or winter snow. However, the power of the music isn't so much in the exact reproduction of the sounds of birds singing or ice cracking. Rather Vivaldi's music evokes the sensation of listening to birds or feeling cold. Furthermore, it's perfectly possible to enjoy *The Four Seasons* without thinking about anything outside the music: not all music necessarily refers directly to things in the outside world. Unlike words, with music it's not about "getting the message," even when the song has lyrics. Something else is going on.

Susanne Langer suggests that the power of music lies in something more subtle than imitation of sounds we encounter elsewhere: a phenomenon she terms "isomorphism": "Patterns of similarity between the structure of the musical rhythms and melodies and the structure of other cognitive, discursive, and above all emotional 'objects' to which music reaches."[8] From Langer's point of view, music does carry meaning, just as language does. But unlike language, music does not represent concepts; rather, it offers a "morphology of feeling from one system of signs to another."[9] We "hear" our feelings, just as Henry hears "love" in the music of Cab Calloway. As Caroll Pratt put it in 1931, in *The Meaning of Music*, music "sounds the way moods feel."[10]

The power of music, then, in Langer's view, lies in its power to evoke feeling while retaining a fundamental ambiguity and ambivalence. Music is an "unconsummated symbol":

> Music has all the earmarks of a true symbolism, except one: the existence of an assigned connotation. It is a form that is capable of connotation, and the meanings to which it is amenable are articulations of emotive, vital, sentient experiences. But its import is never fixed.[11]

The power of music to evoke strong feelings without confining them to specific meanings has enormous practical benefits in dementia care. Sharing an experience that has meaning for the caregiver and for the loved one can be deeply pleasant for both, while releasing their shared experience from the burden of aligning the meaning of the experience between them in language. When the ambiguities of the imagining mode become burdensome, due to an increasingly vague or eccentric use of language and categories, listening to a song or singing it after a fashion can provide a connection.

The Pulse of Music

Music, then, inspires emotions. Can we tell what those emotions are? Music theorists continue to debate whether the emotions are coming from the composer or performer or the listener. But amid the debates, one particularly suggestive thread of discussion deals with a sensation that theorists term "satisfaction."

Satisfaction, or enjoyment, according to the nineteenth-century music critic Eduard Hanslick, is an aesthetic experience based on expectation:

> The most important factor in the psychic process that accompanies the comprehension of a musical work and makes it enjoyable is most frequently overlooked. It is the intellectual gratification that the listener finds in continuously following and anticipating the intentions of the composer, here to have his expectations confirmed, there finding himself pleasantly misled.[12]

Music may inspire joy; it may inspire fear; it may inspire any range of emotions, some inspired by the composer's intention and some stimulated by the experiences of the listener. But above all, it must inspire satisfaction: an appreciation of the inherent skill of execution, an appreciation based on anticipating where the music will go and either having the expectations pleasantly confirmed or pleasantly surprised.

Theorists of music, struggling to find the source of that satisfaction repeatedly come back to the notions of time and movement. For Hanslick, music works through "audible changes in force, motion and proportion."[13] Langer concurs that the enjoyment of music has a dynamic quality to it:

> There are certain aspects of the so-called "inner life" – physical or mental – which have formal properties similar to music – patterns of motion and rest, of tension and release, of agreement and disagreement, preparation, fulfilment, excitation, sudden change, etc.[14]

Langer and Hanslick, among others, locate the appeal of music – its qualities of "satisfaction" – within the passing of time, and the changing of the sounds as the time passes. Music "goes somewhere," and according to Meyer, the satisfaction lies in the listener's ability to follow where the music goes: "one musical event (be it a tone, a phrase, or a whole section) has meaning because it points to and makes us expect another musical event."[15] For Leonard Meyer, the expectation is based on our conditioned acceptance of musical norms: the conventions of musical styles and genres and constructs teach us to expect certain melodic and harmonic progressions, and to feel satisfaction when they happen. For David Huron, the expectation is statistical and arises from regression towards the mean: we expect certain movements to occur because we've come to expect them as "average" outcomes.[16] Either way, music, whether live or recorded, is experienced in time and unfolds according to patterns that are typically anticipated, if not always satisfied. Music can often surprise us by failing to resolve as we expect, by modulating into another key, by introducing dissonances and syncopation that defy our expectations. But according to music theorists, the expectations are there, and our enjoyment hinges on the way we follow from musical moment to musical moment, balancing our expectations against what is actually happening as the music progresses.

Relationship to Caregiving

Satisfaction is by no means limited to music: we find it in any field which requires high levels of precision in construction and deftness in execution. Hence, the famous lyricist Cole Porter paid Stephen Sondheim an unexpected compliment when Sondheim shared his lyrics to the musical *Gypsy* with the dying composer:

> I heard a gasp of delight in the corner of the room. Mr. Porter had been caught by surprise: he hadn't anticipated the quadruple

rhyme. Needless to say, surprising a pro is one of the greatest joys a writer can experience ... it may well be the high point of my lyric-writing life.[17]

And the dying James Baldwin is reported by his biographer breaking into a wide, satisfied smile at a particularly brilliant sentence by Jane Austen and whispering, "So economical. So devastating."[18] Surprising a pro into delight is one thing. Surprising a dying pro into delight brings the achievement to a whole new level. I speak from experience: watching a look of surprised delight animate a face that has appeared vacant and forlorn only moments earlier is a good feeling. On some level, everyone with dementia is a pro at something, and everyone with dementia deserves a delightful surprise.

Whether or not the caregiver actually makes a connection through music, then, the theoretical nature of music's influence provides a deep insight into the nature of caring for a loved one with dementia. First, it provides a metaphor of harmonics to envision different levels of recognition and interaction: one in which there is room for confusion over specifics, while retaining an overarching intimacy. Second, it provides a symbolic language without specific referents, enabling caregiver and loved one to experience mutual enjoyment which is not necessarily the same enjoyment. Third, it extends the experience over a temporal period in which the structures of the music enable the listener to anticipate the movement from one musical figure to the next.

The Caregiver's Responsibility

There's a danger in all of this: a danger of treating activities like music as a massive "Get Out of Jail Free" card. I can mean one thing. Dad can mean something different. And we just toddle along on our parallel paths, neither of us minding what the other has to say. But the qualities of music I've defined here are not simply clues to how the caregiver and the loved one can get along without quarrelling. These qualities suggest the conditions in which the caregiver can try to meet the loved one in a more challenging way. Here's Mike Barnes on the need for meaning:

> Meaning, many would say, is in short supply on a dementia ward. Certainly it often seems so. But the shortage of meaning is not just on the side of the demented. It is on our side too. We, who may mean more as we keep asserting, also mean differently. We demand meaning they can't supply. But they also require meaning we can't supply. And they supply meaning, perhaps in abundance, that we can't recognize because we've never felt the need to ask for it.[19]

The stable connection, the capacity to find different levels of meaning, the ability to enjoy a mutual experience without insisting on both deriving the same literal meaning – all of these features give the caregiver an opportunity to grope for the meaning we frequently are too busy and worried and sad to recognize. It's a meaning that comes from regularly repeated sequences of actions that take the form of ritual, carried out in a state of calm that enables the caregiver to take actual delight in the companionship of the loved one. Ben played cards with his mother. George danced with his mother to the radio. Victor and his father built small robot dinosaurs from kits purchased from Lee Valley Tools. Cathie Borrie learned to revel in the whimsical eccentricity of her mother's conversation. And Heather Menzies provides a vivid example of this connection through the practice of sharing tea with her mother:

Tea on her bed, with those same teacups and the same appreciative comments about them every time, became our regular ritual, and every time it seemed to take on more lustre, more resonance almost, like a melody line in a concerto for piano and violin, offset in infinite variations by first the one and then the other instrument. It resembled too the gestures of approach, retreat, lingering, and longing in a lovers' pas de deux. And increasingly I could just enjoy them for what they were, gestures of our connection. I could dwell in those moments sharing a cup of tea with Mum, and be satisfied.[20]

These are touching moments. But how do they constitute the imaginative mode that I described at the beginning of chapter 9?

Having been trained initially in literary studies, I can't help thinking of all those poems and novels and memoirs I've read that describe special moments of perceptive intensity. The British Romantic poets associated such moments with sublime landscapes like mountains and cliffs and gorges. William Wordsworth called them "spots of time": moments in which our attention is heightened, and the details of an experience are etched into our minds, so that we remember them years later. These intense moments, later recollected in tranquility and put into some aesthetic form, comprise the essence of imaginative writing. Virginia Woolf called them "moments of being," separated from the "cotton wool" of ordinary, everyday perception. When George danced with his mother, and Victor built dinosaurs with his father, and Borrie chatted with her mother about the sky, and Menzies had tea with her mother, were these moments when caregiver and loved one step out of the cotton wool into vivid moments of being?

After some tranquil recollection, I've decided that the answer is no. Something more important is happening: a temporary and precious recovery of the cotton wool of life. As cognitively unimpaired adults, we often take ordinary life for granted; we overlook the rhythmic pulse of day-to-day communal living in the world. By finding it in ourselves to relax and be calm in our loved one's presence, by allowing the conversation to take its repetitive course, by following familiar and established rituals in which both participate, we enable our loved ones to experience "the normal" once again.

The imaginative mode, as I conceive it, needn't be a vision on a mountaintop, like Moses talking to God on Mount Sinai. When a loved one has dementia, sometimes the most precious thing you can give that person is a sense of doing something that was once familiar, but which has now become mysterious. Rituals of daily life – folding laundry, washing dishes, walking to the post office, making tea – can be joyful things for someone who has rediscovered the satisfaction of doing them. The satisfaction can be shared between the loved one, who has recovered a sense of agency and command, and the caregiver, who, under the right circumstances, learns to value such mundane matters in a new way. As Tennyson once put it, extraordinary visions are all very well for the mountaintop, but in the end, love is of the valley.

PART SIX

Closing the Distance

As he goes out, I hear the nurse speaking to him in the corridor.
"She's got an amazing constitution, your mother. One of those hearts that just keeps on working, whatever else is gone."
A pause, and then Marvin replies.
"She's a holy terror," he says.
Listening, I feel like it is more than I could now reasonably have expected out of life, for he has spoken with such anger and such tenderness.
– Margaret Laurence, *The Stone Angel*[1]

PART SIX

Closing the Distance

CHAPTER ELEVEN

A Skeptical Pause

For we all of us, grave or light, get our thoughts entangled in metaphors, and act fatally on the strength of them.

– George Eliot, *Middlemarch*[2]

If you've reached this far into the book, I'm guessing that you found a few things interesting or useful. But I'm also willing to bet that you're feeling some skepticism as well. "OK," I can imagine you saying, "this is a nice little four-part scheme, but I can think of several instances in my own experience which don't fit. And where on earth is it all going? At the end of the day, who cares about modes?"

These are valid questions. No scheme works all the time, and no analogy fits every situation. Every teacher, every mentor, every friend, family, or lover has limits. Even the dog who sleeps by my chair as I write this has limits. If we embrace a theory without question and without hesitation, what started as an empowering exercise turns into another metaphor that entangles us. Patterns and schemes can only play fruitful roles in our lives if we acknowledge and assess those limits. So before I start extolling the possibilities of the four-part modal scheme I've developed in these pages, I want to draw some sketchy outlines of its outer borders: the places where it stops working.

Limitations of the Research

The first set of limits rests firmly on me: on the choices I made and the way I carried them out. This is not an act of original research in medicine or nursing or psychology; it is, rather, an imaginative synthesis of existing research, structured on the principles of literary theory and library classification. The empirical and theoretical research on dementia is enormous, taking place in many different disciplines and using many different research methods. There is more research on dementia than any one person can read, and new research is coming out every month. Whatever value this book has lies not in the discovery of hitherto unknown truth, but in making the different strands of truth-seeking fit together in some harmonious way that is useful for a family caregiver. The aim, as I stated in the earlier chapters, is coherence: a coherence in which the various bodies of research can align with the urgent needs of family caregivers. We need some kind of coherence, I believe, for a relationship between family members to survive when one of them has developed dementia.

The scheme of this book also presupposes a deep and loving bond between the caregiver and the one being cared for. It therefore touches only peripherally on the very different caregiving skills acquired by staff in assisted living facilities. The nurses, administrators, and personal support workers in long-term care centers exhibit skills that demand the profound and unsentimental compassion of service to all those in a community, without discrimination: skills of consistency, competence, accountability, equality, efficiency, and courtesy, which they exercise with very little access to each person's backstory. In this book, we're concerned with the complementary opposite: a deep commitment to one person with whom we share a history.

The scheme also has little to offer those whose relationships with the person with dementia suffer from a long-standing and bitter dysfunction. Long-standing "issues" are one thing: most of us, no matter how much we love someone, have scores that remain unsettled, some minor, some serious. Married couples have gone to their graves in entrenched disagreement about the appropriate thermostat setting; some parents and children bear rancorous memories of earlier quarrels that were long forgiven but never entirely forgotten. Those are things we all share. But if the caregiver's relationship to the family member is scarred with deep wounds, bitter hostilities, and abuses of the sort that make estrangement the only safe option for the relative, I'm not sure that this book has much to offer. I'm writing from the assumption that the caregiver desires to preserve a meaningful emotional connection with the loved one and to allow it to develop and change as the condition progresses.

Another limitation has probably struck you at some point in the reading of the last ten chapters. We hear very little from family members with dementia. There exists a growing corpus of writing by people actually living with dementia, writing that takes many different forms. Authors such as Diana Freel McGowin, Ken Sobol (with the help of his wife Julie Macfie Sobol) and Thomas DeBaggio have written memoirs of their personal experiences; others, such as Jennifer Bute, have used their academic backgrounds to facilitate research in dementia. And beyond such formal publications, there exists a growing number of blogs and vlogs, poems, diaries, and other testaments to the experiences of people living with dementia.

These are important voices, and they will become more important as the stigma of dementia diminishes. The Alzheimer Society of Canada, for instance, has established the Advisory Group of People with Lived Experience of Dementia, to ensure that these voices will assume an important role in the development of services and programs to support people living with dementia.[3] I chose, however, to focus my attention exclusively on the caregivers, out of a sense of urgent obligation to give primacy to their experiences. Caring for a family member with dementia is a momentous experience in its own right, and one that brings its own urgent issues of survival. The demands can place a caregiver's physical and mental health at risk. Others in the caregiver's life – spouses, children, colleagues – exert equally valid claims on their strength. And caregiving raises urgent and profound questions of loyalty and allegiance that we must confront as best we can.

I sincerely hope that by taking measures to understand the caregiving experience in its complexity, and by giving some attention to what caregivers experience, this book will enable caregivers to enhance their listening and empathetic skills. Because the most important communication that persons with dementia can make to their loved ones may well come in the later stages, when formal and conventional communication is no longer possible for them. The airline truism – put your own mask on before assisting others – can be easily abused and twisted into a justification for any amount of selfish behavior. Nonetheless, the analogy holds true in this case: to comprehend the communicative efforts of loved ones with dementia, we have to make sure that we are prepared to receive them. And that requires a certain amount of self-care.

So yes. The book you're reading is based on thoughtful but selective reading of research and memoirs, together with the insights of a small group of dementia caregivers, and all of it filtered implicitly through my own experiences of caring for two parents with differing forms of dementia. It makes no pretense of exhaustiveness. But if I've done it properly, the categories I've defined and arranged provide you, as a caregiver, with room: room for your own experiences to fit, room for your own thoughts to develop, and room for new ways to survive.

Limitations of the Metaphor

The second set of limits rests with the metaphor I chose. This book is using Northrop Frye's four-mode system as an analogy for the different ways available to us for thinking of dementia care. If you've read any of Northrop Frye's books (and they're well worth the read), you know that Frye loved myth. Myth, for Frye, constituted the fundamental underlying structures of human understanding, articulating the central, most basic concerns of being alive in the world. Frye also loved the four seasons; his theory of myths in *Anatomy of Criticism* equates comedy with spring, romance with summer, tragedy with autumn, and irony and satire with winter.[4] Frye loved old things: old stories, ancient wisdom, venerable genres, and enduring motifs.

I like old things too, and I like putting things in order: that's why Frye speaks to me. But this approach can also be very annoying. When we're going through something intense in the here and now, the last thing we need is someone looking very wise on the sidelines and quoting ancient authors and classical analogues. As someone who's habitually quoting favorite authors and TV shows and movies, I learned very early on that sometimes it's wiser simply to shut up and lend a hand.

Furthermore, dementia care does not follow the stately and predictable progression of the seasons. Rather, you have to be ready, as the caregiver, to flip back and forth with almost no warning. You can go to visit your loved one in a nursing home anticipating some pleasant time in the imagining mode, singing old songs, only to confront evidence that the loved one has suffered a severe setback, requiring you to think in the descriptive mode, securing new assessments and new medications and new levels of care. Or your family member has developed a strange new behavior that is disrupting the lives of others, requiring you to switch into understanding mode and pay close and careful attention.

Nor are these modes mutually exclusive. If your loved one exhibits a decline in ability, you need to draw on both the understanding mode to determine the nature and extent of the change and the descriptive mode to understand the doctor's assessment and prescription. If the family member is agitated and causing disruption, you may need to draw on both understanding, to determine the problem, and the advocating mode, if the problem was caused by some unsatisfactory treatment by the staff. Above all, you may be in no condition to sit calmly and sing songs. Even as you strain to leave all your other anxieties and responsibilities outside, you may find yourself unable to calm down and enter the imaginative mode, and you may be persecuting yourself inside for that inability, questioning your own loyalty and devotion.

It's a sad fact for people like me who love classification systems: the systems may be neat, but real life is messy. That's true for pretty much every walk of life and every domain of study. In the case of dementia care, real life is more than messy: it's messy and sad. No amount of helpful categorizing is going to turn dementia care into an easy, fun, and stress-free experience.

Life after Care

This leads us to perhaps the biggest question of all. Do you want dementia care to change your life? As family members, we didn't ask to become caregivers; we're not doing this out of any deep-seated vocation for nursing or eldercare. A few of us might discover such a vocation, to be sure, but for most of us, this is an activity that will last as long we're needed. And after it's over – after the loved one has moved beyond our care – many of us plan to forget the past few years as best we can. Enough of nursing homes; enough of phone calls in the middle of the night, of hospitals, of falls and confusion and incontinence, of angry and abusive tirades, of endless days of fear and guilt and suppressed frustration. Better by far to remember the loved one in the early days: the days of vitality and accomplishment, of travel and laughter and good food and good friends.

Do you want dementia care to change your life? Perhaps not, and that's perfectly fair. Perhaps you have plans, a goal, an objective. There are many good plans and admirable goals, and while others may pass judgment on you from a distance for not being the saint that society expects you to be, you shouldn't let such superficial views affect your own judgment. Perhaps you have other responsibilities: to children, or to your work, or to other important causes. In such cases, you may well reach a firm decision: you will do what you need to do, but these other claims take priority. Dementia care will be something you do, but it will play no role in how you define yourself.

Perhaps, also, you may object to the trite glorifications of the caregiving role. In the DVD commentary to "The Body," his poignant episode of *Buffy the Vampire Slayer* which confronts the mundane realities of death, author and producer Joss Whedon alludes to his mother's death, and expresses staunch resistance to the notion that enduring such sadness makes you a better person.[5] Nuts to that, you may say. I'll survive this experience of dementia care because I have no other choice. But no one, no one is going to tell me that "it's all for the best." As I mentioned in the first chapter of this book, dementia care is not a skill that we master but an experience we survive.

In the following chapter, I'm not going to argue that dementia care makes you a better person. But I AM, however, going to qualify what I said earlier. Beneath all the trite "Never say die" and "It's all for the best" stuff, I am going to argue that, under certain circumstances and with a healthy bit of good luck, dementia care can help you in your broader life. It's just possible that you will emerge on the other side of the experience with some unexpected skills and ways of thinking that are surprisingly resilient and relevant to the general task of living. After you've had a good long rest.

CHAPTER TWELVE

An Optimistic Conclusion

Let's return to the concept of coherence that I raised in the early chapters. Coherence is the aim of this work: taking a complex situation and laying it out in an orderly array. When we've organized a subject coherently, we have the sensation of grasping the entire domain: a sense of cognitive possession of the entire situation. This possession arises from a combination of analysis and synthesis. On the one hand, we separate things into different categories; on the other, we combine these categories into a single well-constructed scheme. This book has aimed to make the general task of family dementia care coherent by separating out the different modes and then linking them together into a sequence.

Why do we need coherence? For one thing, we need it for our own sanity: when we are overwhelmed by the different tasks facing us and the different emotions that each task provokes in us, we need coherence to keep us from freezing into paralysis. We need to find those patterns of regularity that give us at least some means of assessing the present and predicting the future, however vaguely. As Agatha Christie's Hercule Poirot would say, we need order and method to disentangle the knotted clues and figure out what needs to be done. And in that sense, coherence also enables us to provide better, more targeted care.

In addition to keeping our sanity and making us better caregivers, coherence helps us to perform a further act of classification. It enables us to distinguish which skills apply only to the job at hand and which can actually serve us beyond the immediate need. As I hope to show, each mode has its share of benefits, some of which help us survive the present and some which could help us flourish in the future.

The Descriptive Mode

In the earlier chapters, I discussed the way in which the medical establishment treats dementia as something "abnormal": as a condition that is not part of "normal aging." It's a problematic distinction in many ways, but at the same time, there's something releasing about it for the caregiver. In those treacherous early days, where the symptoms are insidiously appearing here and there like strange ripples on the surface of daily life, the loved one's family is frequently at a loss, or worse, at odds with each other. Am I imagining things? Am I making too much of these strange bouts of absent-mindedness, or signs of depression, or failures to remember familiar words? Some family members might say yes, while others might say no; we might say yes on Monday, and then reverse ourselves on Tuesday. The diagnosis, harsh as it may be, releases us from at least some of that frantic second-guessing. Whatever is going on, at least we can be sure that it's not all in our head. *Something* real is going on, and that frees us to grapple with it out in the open.

I also mentioned the terminological complexity of the descriptive mode: the many kinds of dementia, the confusion over the causes, the difficulty of reaching an accurate diagnosis. This too can be frustrating: the stark results of a failed cognition test blossom into many-branched considerations, where no one, it seems, can give us a straight answer, and every expert in every field appears to be madly hedging bets. On the other hand, the proliferation of terms in the descriptive mode, and our growing awareness of the nuances of dementia that comes from learning them, releases us from the brutality of inherited popular conceptions of dementia as a curse and a disgrace: a form of insanity that terrifies us.

Once you start digging into the research on dementia, you can experience other forms of freedom. Whether you're researching the condition itself, nursing and care practices, or the policy implications of caring for people on a global, national, or local level, you start to notice some interesting things.

First and foremost, it's not just you. That may seem obvious, but it's something we all need to remember, especially if we've inherited an entrenched tradition of regarding dementia as a shameful family secret to be hidden away and dealt with behind closed doors. Many, many people are dealing with family members with dementia, all over the world. What's more, many people are dealing with it in our own communities, and often they are willing to share insights, share findings, share experiences.

There are also many people trying to help. Researchers from multiple fields are converging on dementia, ranging from large, multidisciplinary research alliances to small, specialized studies, and examining many different aspects of dementia and dementia care. In my own field of information studies and knowledge organization, for instance, there is a growing interest in ways that big data and artificial intelligence can be used to solve some of the pressing problems of dementia care, including finding more accurate predictors of dementia so that the treatment can begin earlier.[1] On a smaller scale, libraries are actively researching how to participate in and facilitate community-based dementia care through their collections and programming.[2] These are just two examples of research that extend beyond medical research in the strictest sense, providing ideas, suggestions, and future directions for testing in all aspects of dementia care.

Here's where the descriptive mode carries hidden benefits beyond dementia care. When you immerse yourself in the empirical research around dementia, you get an insight into how we increase our knowledge of the world. I don't mean simply knowledge of dementia, or even medicine: I mean knowledge of all kinds of things. When I was growing up, I learned in school about "the scientific method," with its seven steps of empirical research: question, research, hypothesis, experiment, data analysis, conclusion, and communication. At the time, it didn't mean much to me: it seemed far, far away from the problems that obsessed me as a high school student, and in later years I got into the humanities with its different research paradigms. But researching dementia in the scientific literature provides a view of human understanding that I find fascinating and strangely moving: all the more so because it's so different from the way we see it working in movies.

Goodness knows, the research in all those journal articles isn't glamorous; sometimes it's barely readable. But when you look at the research studies in dementia, you see a research tradition that is committed to skepticism and resistance to quick, easy answers. You see entrenched mechanisms for checking and verifying and querying and enhancing and qualifying the findings of others. You see knowledge emerging through collaborative effort, across language barriers and cultural barriers and geographical barriers. You witness bravery, courage, and determination: not focused on a single heroic individual who challenges "the establishment," but distributed across a wide community of conscientious researchers who insist on showing up to a problem, often for years on end.

There's a lot wrong with empirical research, of course: every field is littered with missed opportunities, overlooked insights, mistakes and false starts, not to mention all the prejudice and blindness that occur when human beings try to work together. But I find this copious outpouring of research inspiring. It may not make good cinema, but whether you follow the research directly, or through mediating sources like journalists who distil the findings for the general public, or through the services of Alzheimer societies, you may find it inspiring a response you never thought you'd have in a caregiving situation: curiosity. Even after you've closed the book and shredded all your notes on dementia, you may find that your capacity to be intrigued at what you don't know, and your ability to ask questions without being intimidated, has stayed with you. If so, it can't hurt.

The Understanding Mode

When it comes to understanding how the world looks from the perspective of the person with dementia, a close family member has a significant edge over the various doctors, nurses, and support workers who provide care. As family members, we know the person and have typically known them for years. We know their history: in particular, we know of specific events that were meaningful, transformative, or traumatic. We can connect the loved one's sadness on a particular day with the anniversary of someone's death. We can explain to a baffled care worker that the person used to run a care home herself, which is why she tends to grab a clipboard and walk up and down the halls of the care center giving orders to the staff. We know what the loved one is like if woken from an afternoon nap; we know that the loved one reacts badly to scary movies; we know that strawberries and cream are the greatest treats imaginable and that the photos on the sideboard are images of precious children and grandchildren. We know what music the loved one likes, along with favorite TV shows and preferred clothing styles.

As the dementia progresses, however, this edge can turn against the caregiver. Signs of neglect begin to appear, as the loved one starts to abandon a lifelong interest that is growing beyond their capacity. The knitting bag gathers dust in a corner. Favorite books languish on the shelves. A favorite TV show provokes restlessness and boredom. The photos on the sideboard inspire no visible emotion, or even recognition.

In addition to neglect, we often see signs of change, and sometimes these changes startle us. A mother who spent the last ten years watching Miss Marple suddenly takes a fancy to science fiction movies; a father who played classical music all his life starts tapping his feet enthusiastically to country music. And residents in a nursing home often find new friends and intimate attachments: sometimes with people we never expected. André Maurois once noted that in literature, as in love, we are astonished at the choices of others. It holds as true in nursing homes as it does at high school proms.

These changes can feel like a betrayal. They can tempt us to "freeze" our helpless loved ones in a form of stasis and insist that they continue to be the loved one of old: surrounded by books they can no longer read, music that no longer moves them, clothes that no longer fit, and food that no longer agrees with them. In such situations, we can't help but measure the person by a yardstick of decline, seeing an ever-expanding gap between the person they were and the person they are.

Here is where the understanding mode comes to our aid. In this mode, we exert our listening and observational powers to understand, as best we can, how the world appears from the loved one's perspective. This is particularly important in sensitive topics, such as sexuality. Only in the understanding mode is a caregiver able to cope with the delicate negotiations necessary for recognizing how sexuality and sexual identity frequently continue and frequently change in dementia situations.[3] In so doing, we recognize that concrete changes are taking place in the person's powers of conversation, as well as in the person's ability to categorize and name the people and things and emotions that mark the progress of living in the world. And however sad these changes may be, by following them we are able to continue learning, and our relationship with our loved ones continues to grow and develop.

Extended contact with a loved one with dementia leads us away from certainties about someone we know very well. Dementia does not make a person simpler; it makes a person more mysterious. It's daunting, sometimes, to realize how little we really know about the entire life of someone, even someone close to us. The spouse with whom we celebrated a golden anniversary had a life before marriage; the mother who gave birth to us had a life before we came along. As their power to convey coherent information about that life diminishes, we are left with many unanswered questions.

When we listen and watch closely as our loved ones struggle to adapt to changes taking place within their bodies and outside them, we honor them by bearing witness. We learn how these changes are affecting them and become better able to understand their efforts to reach out to us. And we see, increasingly, that these people we've known for so long are, ultimately, secrets to us. Such a recognition can inspire a response you never thought to feel as a caregiver: awe. In the impassivity of the loved one's face, and in the faint suggestions here and there of past incidents and experiences about which we knew nothing, we wonder at the mysteries that hover around another person, even one we've loved for years.

The Advocating Mode

A lot of unpleasant thoughts come up in the advocating mode: difficult questions that we ask of caregivers, of other family members and of ourselves. Where are your loyalties? What is your allegiance? At the end of the day, who are you *really* trying to serve? Ugly thoughts can reach the light of day, as caregivers wrestle with nightmarish fears on both grand and small scales. Is my loved one being abused in a chamber of horrors? Is my loved one being cheated by smiling faces that profess to be devoted but who are merely self-serving? Are my family and children truly helping me as much as they can? Worst of all, am I, myself, *honestly* doing all I can possibly do?

No one wants those nightmares. Working through them, however, can release the caregiver into some unexpected states of freedom. As we learn more and more about health care systems and assisted living conditions and the social support structures available to us, we gradually gain clarity about the things we need to fight for and the things we can let slide. We may decide, for instance, that our lonely and gregarious loved one can cope with sharing a room, but that dietary needs must be met exactly; we may be willing to accept a facility's entertainment offerings but ask penetrating questions about access to exercise and fresh air.

In asking these questions, caregivers add clarity to their own obligations and needs: they are better able to make reasonable assessments of the toll that caregiving is taking on them and on their various other obligations. Ideally, these assessments enable frank discussions with other family members about sharing of tasks. They also enable the caregiver to make reasonable requests for accommodation from employers and sensible applications for government services.

Rarely are any of these conversations free of stress, and not all of them are successful. Not all employers are sympathetic; not all regions have access to a wide range of community services. Some situations are wretched through and through. Above all, not all families are functional, and even the most loving family might need to work hard to mend breaches in the years that follow. Nonetheless, in many cases, learning to choose one's battles and articulate one's needs can serve to release families from the vague realm of guilt expiation. Having frank and honest discussions about requirements and needs can enable those family members at a greater remove to spend less time and energy battling their guilt and spending more time figuring out ways of supporting from a distance. Caregivers on the ground can likewise spend less time resenting those who seem to be defaulting on their duty and more time on providing workable and realistic suggestions.

The advocating mode, then, is a difficult but important mode of thinking and acting and problem-solving during the period of dementia care. But what about afterwards?

If you're currently caring for a family member with dementia, advocacy tends to be concentrated on the loved one: in a bad situation, we are looking out for our own. But even in the thick of caregiving, we witness the broader picture, even if we haven't the immediate energy to address it directly. Elder care in Canada, as elsewhere, is in a deeply vulnerable situation, especially since the COVID pandemic. We can rarely watch the news without seeing stories of our aging population, of the reduction of government oversight over retirement and long-term care facilities, of overworked care workers fighting off burnout. And we must never forget what it feels like, during an outbreak of infection, to stand outside locked-down care homes, as our baffled and frightened loved ones looked at us through windows: at least those relatives who were well enough to stand or sit.

Clearly, there is room for advocacy in the more general sense of the term: bringing our energy and time and voices to bear on behalf of a broader group of individuals who need assistance in fighting for their needs and rights. Government services, both to persons with dementia and their caregivers, must be maintained and improved. Government standards and regulations for retirement homes and long-term care facilities must be maintained. Libraries and community centers must continue to involve themselves in improving the quality of life for those living with dementia. Research must continue.

As family caregivers, we have learned certain things that governments, researchers, and health care systems need to remember:

- You cannot disguise inadequate care by dressing it up in the false luxury of a cruise ship;
- Dementia care requires close and productive cooperation between the personal care of family members and the general care of health care systems;
- Well-trained, decently paid, and dedicated health care workers of all kinds, in sufficient numbers, are absolutely essential to any society that professes to care for its more vulnerable citizens;
- Caring for its vulnerable citizens is the hallmark of a society worth preserving.

An Optimistic Conclusion 177

After your loved one has moved beyond your personal care, you may feel an unexpected emotion: a desire to work for broader change and to challenge your government and your community to address the problems that you experienced so viscerally when you were fighting for one person. If that happens, rest assured: there is much to do.

The Imaginative Mode

In my chapters on the imaginative mode, I expressed some skepticism towards the "miracle cure" approach to the creative arts in dementia care: I wasn't sure it was wise to invest too heavily in the notion that music made people shed their dementia like magic, or that it was necessarily and inevitably a great experience for the person with dementia or the family caregiver. That said, there is lots of interesting work to be done on how the creative arts might play a role in the lives of people living with dementia. Following the lead of Anne Davis Basting, there is more we can learn about the interaction of people who live with dementia with creative activities of all sorts. And the research of cognitive psychologist and neuroscientist Daniel Levitin suggests that we are on the threshold of new discoveries about the ways in which music affects the brain:

> The study of human behavior has undergone a revolution in the past twenty years, as the methods of neuroscience have been applied to cognition and the musical experience. We can now actually see the brain at work, mapping those regions that are active during certain activities.[4]

Given the popularity of Levitin's work and the rising interest among researchers in this area, we can expect some interesting research to emerge in the next few years.[5]

In the meantime, it's worth remembering what the arts give us, generally, as human beings. And one of the greatest gifts is a structured place to play and enjoy ourselves. Dante appeased the anxiety of his readers, lost in the dark woods of life, by guiding them through a set of carefully constructed landscapes, each explained by a guide. As Alfred Hitchcock explained to readers of *Good Housekeeping* in 1949, the regular conventions and procedures of motion pictures enable people to experience vicarious fear "without paying the price."[6] Aristotle used the term *catharsis* to denote the way we purge ourselves of emotions like pity and fear through watching a tragedy.[7] We enjoy activities and rituals that arouse our emotions and sensations within safe and bounded domains, dominated by regular and recognizable traditions and procedures. And while the arts have articulated these principles and cultivated the intense skills of executing them, they don't hold the patent on the satisfaction we can feel in dementia caregiving. The sensations aroused need not be the mighty ones of fear or pity. They can be as simple and basic as enjoying a familiar cup of tea, recognizing a familiar teacup, or smiling at a familiar face, even when the name won't surface in the memory.

Sharing moments of safe and structured connection with a loved one living with dementia can be a profound experience, for two reasons. First, it can amaze us sometimes, that in the rush and upheaval of dementia care, we find ourselves actually enjoying ourselves, living in the present, without a pressing sense of urgency or worry or exhaustion. Second, such moments retain a certain mystery, a mystery embodied in the fact that we often don't fully grasp the nature of the connection between ourselves and the person with whom we're sharing that special moment. Because the connection may be taking place on different levels: consistent and harmonious, but different. As with the describing mode, the understanding mode, and the advocating mode, the imagining mode leaves the caregiver with unanswered questions and evidence that appears to point in more than one direction. In that sense, the caregiver's analysis resembles Roger Scruton's comparison of finding meaning in music to seeing a face in the clouds:

> Consider the face in the cloud. You see the face in the cloud only when you also see that it is not there. To believe that there is a face in the cloud is not (in the relevant sense) to perceive it. It is to be the victim of an illusion ... There is a transfer involved in seeing the face: the intentional object of experience must be described using a concept that is known not to apply to the material object of perception.[8]

In the imaginative mode, the caregiver chooses to see a face in the cloud: a choice based on a patient and loving exposure to the loved one and a desire to frame the loved one in a pattern that we may not entirely believe but choose to accept. This is one of those moments where two opposed statements are true. In so doing, the caregiver may feel an unexpected sensation: one of irony.

Sensations of curiosity about the things we don't know. Awe at the mysteries we encounter in ordinary life. Commitment to making positive change in the world. Savoring a paradox that lies at the heart of many a quiet moment. None of these will shield us from any malign twists of fate that lie ahead for us. But they may help us survive them. And if so, our loved ones, by receiving our care, may have done us one last, vital service.

EPILOGUE

Learning from an Organist

My mother was an accomplished pianist and organist, and my sisters and I grew up listening not only to Bach and Beethoven but also to the many technical exercises that she used daily, to keep her hands and fingers limber and ready for duty. Whenever I was home sick from school, I would lie in bed listening to those complex and rapid exercises as she moved up and down the octaves. I would try to isolate the recurring patterns and the subtle variations between them. Bach was her favorite composer, and at intervals she would go into one of her "Bach fits," where she would play Bach almost nonstop for one or two days. I remember her once saying happily, "I thought I'd feel guilty neglecting my family and devoting my life to my music. But I don't find it difficult at all."

Like many pianists and organists, Mom was in constant demand to accompany musicians on the piano, play for funerals, and fill in for vacationing church organists. She took these tasks in her stride and with a mordant sense of humor: once, during a particularly busy month of funerals, she put down the phone and remarked, "Another one. They're dropping like flies." Nonetheless, she took the task of supporting musicians very seriously, and one of her favorite books was forever lying open around the house: Gerald Moore's *Am I Too Loud? Memoirs of an Accompanist*.

After Mom died, following a ten-year battle with some combination of Alzheimer's disease and primary progressive aphasia, I had occasion to look through Moore's memoirs myself, and I was intrigued by the parallels between the professional accompanist and the family caregiver. Moore's description of a good accompanist cites many of the skills that family caregivers develop as they support their family members through the stages of dementia:

> [The accompanist] listens sensitively to his singer's voice until he knows its potentialities as well as he knows those of his own pianoforte, giving his partner as much support as he possibly can but at the same time taking care not to overpower or cover the voice.[1]

Family caregivers, when on their game, listen with the same sensitivity, assessing what the loved one is capable of doing and what they as caregivers are capable of supporting.

While a professional lifetime supporting solo artists might seem thankless, Moore was quick to emphasize that true support is not a matter of withdrawing into the background, but rather stepping forward to participate in the central activity. Moore saw the art of accompanying musicians as one of deep engagement. In discussing one of the earliest of the many singers he accompanied, Moore states the following:

> To [Coates] the accompanist was a partner sharing equally with him the mood of the composer. Joy, sadness, passion, exultation, serenity, rage, must be experienced by each of them. The accompanist should be a source of inspiration, and his playing must

shine out in the marvellous introductions and postludes he has to perform.[2]

The "servitude" of the accompanist, it seems, is a deeply creative act. Only by immersing oneself in the music, by rising to meet it with the utmost passion and skill, can the accompanist truly support the soloist. What an irony, I thought, when I read that passage. Only by meeting the soloist with a musical engagement of equal conviction can the accompanist genuinely support the star. Only by truly giving one's all can the accompanist successfully stay out of the way. And that's not a bad way to train for dementia care.

I had an opportunity to witness the connection between caregiving and accompaniment when I attended my mother's final church service as a professional organist. She was filling in as a supply organist at St. Mark's Anglican Church in Niagara-on-the-Lake. Both she and the family knew that this would be her last gig, by her own choice.

Anglican services are far more musically intricate than those of the United Church to which Mom was accustomed, but she had done such services before, and she was prepared. In the half hour before the service, I watched as she took the choir through a brief rehearsal; the aphasia, which at times made her all but incoherent, was nowhere in evidence, and she directed the small but happy group of singers with ease and good humor. She then disappeared up into the organ loft, and the service went off without a hitch. As always with Anglican services, I spent the whole time fumbling with the prayer book trying to figure out where we were and what I was supposed to say. But the organ accompaniment to the service suffered no such fumbling: the music led us securely from one step to the next, and the congregation worshipped calmly. To the best of my knowledge, no one in the congregation knew this was her last service.

After the benediction, as the congregation was gathering up and leaving, I was greeted by an old school companion. I answered his genial inquiries as best I could, while listening to the organ postlude. It was, as I anticipated, Brahms's Choral Prelude Number 3: "O World, I Must Leave Thee."

Years earlier, Mom had showed me the music to this piece, which she was enthusiastically studying with her organ teacher. She showed me how the music was structured as a gradual process of coming to terms with death: how the smooth opening builds in an intensity of anguished denial and resistance until it pauses for a moment of suspension, and then moves into a glorious resolution of acceptance, rather like a baseball player sliding into home plate, and ending on a sustained major chord.

After it was over, Mom stayed in the organ loft out of sight for some time, while I waited for her down below. I'd come to the service to support her, aware of her growing cognitive difficulties and her increasing vulnerability. I don't remember what I was thinking as I sat waiting for her: my mind was all over the place in those early days. Looking back on the experience now, I'm struck by the reversal of roles. The act of worship is, in many ways, a mundane process: people gather on a regular basis to take part in predictable sequences of words and songs and actions. When executed properly, however, the mundane process takes on a special quality, as if the normality of life is rendered back to us with a special elegance and clarity that refreshes us. When caring for someone with dementia, we try, whenever possible, to bring our loved ones into a refreshed state of normality, whether it means sharing a cup of tea or having an idle conversation while watching the birds. It occurs to me now that during that service, the person with dementia was able to summon up sufficient resources from a lifetime of musical training and accompanying experience to sustain the rest of us, largely oblivious, in a brief period of refreshed normality.

When Mom finally emerged, she was composed and cheerful. I told her how well the service had gone, instinctively emphasizing the smooth transitions of the music throughout the service, and how everything in her choice and execution of the music had gone to support the tone and spirit of the worship.

"Good," she said, looking gratified. Then she turned briskly. "Let's get home. Your father will be wanting his lunch."

APPENDIX I

Researching Dementia as a Family Caregiver

Dementia is a maddening thing to witness at close quarters, because aspects of it are darned interesting. If it were happening to someone other than a person we love, it might well be something we want to spend more time studying. As it is, you might find yourself wanting to do more research, if not during the care process, then later. Heather Menzies devoted time after her mother's death to follow up on some persistent questions: time that led to the publication of *Enter Mourning*. Alternatively, you might find the empirical research soothing in its appeal to emotions other than lamentation and its ability to place your experience on a more impersonal basis, if only for a while. If either of these scenarios applies to you, you might want to do more research. Here are some suggestions for following up on what the research community is doing in dementia care.

Be Active, Not Passive!

I know programs like ChatGPT are turning information retrieval into a question-and-answer process which feels a good deal easier than the old-fashioned techniques of looking things up. But for something as important as dementia care, it's important to take control, and sometimes that involves searching, and not just asking. Feeding content to eyeballs is big business in these days of social media, and the impact of artificial intelligence is only going to make that worse. Be careful of information that is "fed" to you through social media feeds: their final aim is to catch your attention and to keep you scrolling. And unfortunately, only certain kinds of information tend to arrest our attention when scrolling through our phones on the bus, and they often tend to arouse anger, shock, and depression.

It's impossible to avoid all the content that's fed to us through newsfeeds and AI summaries on search engines. But try to introduce some method and initiative into searching: start by articulating what you're curious about at the moment, and decide on a source you consider most likely to tell you what you want to know. And if it doesn't work the first time, change your strategy and try again; each time we modify our search, we learn a little bit more about the topic and ourselves and what we want. It may be slower, but it's amazing how a little planning and a sense of purpose can help you find things that are useful.

Sources of Research

As a starting point, I have a crush on a resource called *Medline Plus*, from the US National Library of Medicine. It provides an index of health conditions; for each condition, it gives a short summary of the condition and the chief issues, links to major associations that deal with it, and links to relevant articles in *PubMed*, the Library's major research database. In addition, *Medline Plus* offers an index of Drugs and Supplements, as well as a medical encyclopedia and information on major medical tests.

Of the many databases out there, Google Scholar is by far the easiest and most accessible. It works just like Google: you get a box; you type something into the box; stuff happens. And like Google, the useful stuff in Google Scholar has an eerie way of floating to the top where you can find it easily. Unfortunately, a lot of the stuff that you find in Google Scholar ends up being behind a paywall, unless you're using it in a public or university library that subscribes to all the journals that it searches.

If you want to go further, you might see if your library has access to the following databases:

The Descriptive Mode

For this mode, I recommend *PubMed*, which consists of a massive collection of citations from respected medical journals, together with citations for additional books and full text for some materials selected by the US National Library of Medicine.

The Understanding Mode

Much of the research for the understanding mode comes from the field of psychology. PsycInfo is a database created by the American Psychological Association, containing citations for authoritative research in psychology and the social sciences. You typically need to get it through a library or some other institution; it can also be complex to use, depending on the interface the institution uses.

The Advocating Mode

I recommend two databases here, depending on what you need. If you're looking at standards of care in nursing homes, I'd recommend the *CINAHL* database for nursing and allied health literature. Again, you need to use it through a library's subscription. If you're more concerned with the policy aspects of institutional care, I'd recommend the PAIS (Public Affairs Information Service) Index, which provides access to research in government, health conditions, human rights and politics, public affairs, and social policy.

Filtering Search Results

In all of these databases, keep an eye on ways to filter the search results. Frequently, you can tell the system to limit the findings to a particular language, which is very useful, since dementia research takes place all over the world. You can also often limit by date, which can help if you're looking only for the most recent materials: dementia research has been taking place for a long time.

Some systems allow you to select the *kind* of material you want, and it's worth paying attention to the various options available. Books, of course, can be very helpful, as long as they're up to date and as long as you've got the time to read them. Keep an eye on book reviews as well: if you encounter a book on Amazon that claims to have solved every conceivable problem a home carer could confront, a good book review can help you decide whether or not to give the author a chance to prove those extravagant claims.

Articles come in mainly three categories, each of which is useful. Journal articles from refereed periodicals are the best place to find the tangible research results. Magazine articles provide more simplified and accessible treatments of specific subjects; newspapers report things of current interest.

Hard-core empirical research has very little entertainment value; it's written not for the general public but for others who are researching the same thing, and as such they use terminology most of us don't understand and spend pages and pages documenting and verifying the quality of their methods and the validity of their findings. Fortunately, however, empirical research has a standard structure which most studies adhere to, making it fairly easy to pick out the parts of the article we're likely to understand. I recommend concentrating on these sections:

- The **abstract**: it summarizes the article in one paragraph, giving you an idea of what the researchers were trying to do, how they went about it, and what they found.
- The **introduction**: the first section of an article is usually in accessible language and gives you a sense of the context of the research: how it fits in with what others in the research community are discussing.
- The **findings**: findings can be difficult to understand, especially in quantitative studies that deal largely with measurement and statistical analysis, but it's worth a try. In qualitative studies that are typically more linguistic in nature, the findings are easier to interpret.
- The **discussion**: this is the important part, where the authors draw conclusions from their findings.
- The **limitations**: honest researchers take great care with this section. No study can provide definitive, lasting, eternal certainty, and it's helpful to know the degree of certainty and also the degree to which they can be generalized to a larger population.

Pearl Growing

Often, when we're searching, we don't really know what we're looking for until we find something that clicks. If you happen to find something that's pure gold, use it to find other things of similar value. There are numerous ways of doing this:

- Look at the article's list of citations. Researchers don't pull their brilliance out of a hat; they draw on the brilliance of others. The bibliography shows us who these brilliant people are.
- See who has cited the article. In Google Scholar, there's an easy link called "Cited by" that takes you to others who have used this article.
- Sometimes, the database you're using offers suggestions for similar articles.

Parting Advice

1. **Stop When You Need To.** Dementia research is massive and complex, and you're not using it to cure dementia but merely to survive the experience of witnessing it. As long as the research interests you, empowers you, makes you curious, and suggests alternatives you think worth pursuing in your care, then by all means, go for it.
   And if you're burying yourself in the research in order to deny, or evade, or deflect the sad things pressing on your mind: that's OK too. We all need to hide from the tough stuff from time to time, and if you need the escape, take the escape. Rest assured, the brute necessities will find you sooner or later.

But if the research is baffling you, depressing you, exhausting you, or making you miserable: stop. This is not a school project, and there are no grades.
2. **Decide: Do You Want Information or Affirmation?**
If you've already made up your mind on something – that the medical establishment is corrupt, that Alzheimer's Disease is caused by exposure to a particular substance, or that a particular cognition test is unreliable – admit it up front. Any searching you do will not be a search for information but for a voice that agrees with you. There's nothing inherently wrong with that: goodness knows, I seek out friends who are most likely to amplify and support whatever mood I'm in at the moment. But don't confuse it with genuine information seeking, least of all systematic research. No matter how much time you spend at your laptop – and finding someone who actually agrees with us can sometimes take time – unless you're prepared to expand your view or change your mind in light of new evidence, you're looking for friends and allies, not information.
3. **Be Skeptical, Even When Things Appear to Make Sense.**
Take everything you read, even from sources you trust, with a big lump of rock salt. The best researchers in the world can only provide partial answers to life's mysteries, and if they have integrity, they'll admit that up front. No study tells the whole story. And as Oscar Wilde once put it, even the best of us can be foolish or wrong from time to time.

As for "untrustworthy" sources in this age of Fake News, there are two things that raise red flags for me. The first is the "miracle cure." As you've probably gathered from reading this book, I don't believe in instant, effortless solutions, especially when they appear to come from a single individual who stands in defiance of the medical establishment owing to bravely "thinking outside the box." There's lots wrong with medicine, as with everything else, but I tend to trust collective efforts of conscientious researchers over someone who plays prophet.

The second is the conspiracy theory. I'm sure there are conspiracies here and there, although the ones I've ever witnessed were pretty pathetic affairs. I guess that's why I'm rarely able to take them seriously, in medicine or anywhere else. Human cowardice, stupidity, and crass selfishness, in my opinion, leave the most sinister conspirator with very little harm left to do.

APPENDIX 2

More about Modes

In the main body of the book, I have kept my own experiences as a caregiver to a minimum, confining them to the Preface and Conclusion. However, this book rests firmly upon those personal experiences and the efforts I took to make sense of them, and I feel some obligation to bring them into the light. I'm a scholar and an academic: when faced with stress, my first reaction is to retreat into research. That doesn't always make me the most effective caregiver, but it did lead me into some interesting places that, when combined with my direct experiences with my parents, ultimately led me to write this book. This appendix briefly summarizes some of my research into the theory of modes and how it connected with my own personal caregiving experiences.

Modes

The *Oxford English Dictionary* offers many definitions of the term "mode," and I found two particularly helpful. A mode is "a way or manner in which something is done or takes place; a method of proceeding in any activity, business, etc." It is also "a particular form, manner, or variety in which some quality, phenomenon, or condition occurs or is manifested." As defined here, a mode describes something, but describes it in a very "active" way, as a "way of being."[1] This feels odd at first: it's like saying "my teacup is by way of being blue," which is hardly how we describe a blue teacup these days. But the term is used in various disciplines to describe some form of approach: a way of "closing in" on what is desired from a particular direction, and using particular methods.

My first exposure to the notion of "modes" came in a political philosophy course in my first year as an undergraduate student at University of Toronto. We were studying Plato's *Republic*, and I was startled to read that Socrates, in imagining his ideal society, advised strict rules on the kinds of music allowed. Music in the "mixed Lydian mode" apparently doesn't encourage people to be brave and warlike, but rather to be soft and idle, and should therefore be excluded.[2] This struck me as absurd: what could it possibly matter what people listened to? This banning of certain modes also fed my growing sense that I wouldn't want to live in this "ideal republic." I imagined myself doing endless exercises in a gymnasium against a steady background of military marches.

In later years, however, I came to realize that there were certain kinds of music I can't listen to if I want to get any work done. Some composers that I deeply admire possess an eerie power to drain me of all desire to work and have to be banished from my office. Other kinds of music tend to surface when I'm walking, still others when I'm at the gym, and when I'm doing housework, it's nonstop Broadway. Perhaps Socrates had the right idea after all. Music does affect our emotions, and our emotions affect our moods and actions. And when I found myself caring for two parents with dementia, the concept of the "mode" first became meaningful to me in the context of music.

Modes in Music

Being a violinist, I conducted regular music sessions at my mother's nursing home. These were popular events, and the residents clearly enjoyed singing, not to mention dancing, tapping their feet and chatting with someone outside the facility. Given how dull life can be in a nursing home, I attributed my popularity largely to the novelty. One occasion, however, felt different. The session had been unexpectedly cancelled for some reason, and since I was already there, I took out my violin in the first-floor lounge and began playing softly. A resident I'd never seen before was sitting nearby, motionless and silent. After some moments I witnessed tears welling in his eyes and then running down his face. He never moved; he never spoke; he never turned his head to look at me or to look about him. But the evidence was very strong. Clearly, music has a powerful and mysterious effect on the emotions.

The concept of modes in Western music, however, suggests that it's no great mystery. Take the seven notes that constitute a major scale: they're arranged in a predictable and fixed set of whole- and half-tones. If you start your scale on the bottom of those seven notes, you get the "Ionian" mode, and you can thunder out the theme to *Star Wars* in all its martial glory. If you start it on the second note, the half-tones come in different places, and you have the "Dorian" mode with its air of pensiveness and melancholy, popular in English folk music, as well as in Simon and Garfunkel's "Scarborough Fair/Canticle." All the modes use the seven-note diatonic scale, which Carol Williams calls "the scaffolding of music,"[3] but each makes it sound different, and each has its own emotional connotations.

What was in that man's mind as he sat quietly weeping as I played nearby? He never told me, and I'll never know. Some might suggest that the melody was something familiar from his childhood and that it aroused long lost memories. Some might speculate that the man was once a violinist, or loved a violinist, and reacted to the sound of the instrument. Neurologists might describe the documented effects of music on the brain. But as I pondered the effect of music, not just on that man but on all the residents, I began to gravitate to a simpler working theory. Perhaps the song I was playing combined the full tones and half tones into a mode that made certain emotions available for the man to experience and express. If so, I hope he felt better for it. At any rate, I found myself more and more thinking about mode in relation to dementia and dementia care. Soon I spread beyond music to see how mode is treated in other fields of study. And my next stop lay in the field of language and grammar.

Modes in Grammar

As my parents' dementia progressed, I found myself increasingly exasperated by the loss of nuance in their speech. In making arrangements for their care, my sisters and I were anxious to consult their wishes and were increasingly unable to tell what those wishes were. And some of that had to do with grammar.

In grammar, the term "mode" is typically equated with "mood": a grammatical expression of an attitude that permeates a particular statement, often reflected in either the conjugation of the verb or the inflection of the voice. Assertions frequently use the indicative mode, as in "I did the dishes." Orders take the imperative mode – "Do the dishes" – while statements of doubt or possibility or desire typically take the subjunctive mode: "It might be nice if someone did the dishes."[4]

Grammatical modes enable us to invest our statements with emotions such as certainty, doubt, interrogation, and speculation. Many of us become very good at displacing them for effect. My mother would sometimes give orders in a tone of joyful exclamation. "You could make your bed!" she would cry cheerfully, making it sound as if we'd just won the Lottery. My father sometimes used the subjunctive to express keen irritation: "It would be very nice if you kids could remember to fill the gas tank after you've used the car." Experience tells us what people actually mean through their use of modes. When your boss appears behind you and says quietly, "It would be much appreciated if you finished that report as soon as possible," experience tells you whether the statement truly expresses the doubt, possibility, or desire typical of the subjunctive mode, or whether the boss is using the subjunctive as a mask for an imperative. One is a friendly nudge; the other is a veiled threat. And getting along in a human community often requires us to tell the difference.

My sisters and I found ourselves tripping over our own experience, as our lifelong habits of reading our parents' moods through their grammatical modes became more and more useless. In trying to tell whether Dad was reconciled to giving up the car, whether they liked their new apartment, whether they were happy, whether they trusted us or approved of what we were doing for them, we parsed their statements frantically for nuances that were no longer there.

Modes in Literary Studies

On the day my father died, I returned to my office after my morning class to find a phone message calling me home to Toronto urgently. I quickly arranged a seat on the next train out of London, and while I was boarding, my phone rang. It was my sister, telling me that they could take measures to keep Dad alive until I got there, if I wanted. While putting my coat in the overhead bin and fumbling for my seat, I told her that I'd said my goodbyes to him a few days earlier, and that they needn't take any extreme measures to keep him alive on my account. As I was shouting this over the din of the train, people were streaming past me in the aisle, and the woman next to me had her nose buried in her magazine, straining not to pay attention. The whole scene had a farcical air, and after I was settled in my seat and the train was moving, I thought to myself, "My father's dying, and this wasn't how I imagined it." It felt like the wrong mode: in this case, the wrong *literary* mode.

In literary studies, theorists since Aristotle have used the term "mode" to indicate a specific approach to a genre. Epics like *The Odyssey* are typically approached through poetic narration, while tragedy typically takes place in plays on the stage. Literature, like music, can say all kinds of different things, and evoke all kinds of different emotions. And just as certain musical modes are congenial to specific genres of music, so certain literary modes support certain genres of literature. Think of the difference between a summer action movie and an autumn prestige movie that's aiming for an Oscar nomination. Think of all the different means, from the promotional preview and the movie poster to the choice of music, scenic design, the length, and the cast, that cue us to expect a certain genre of movie. We can define "mode" as that set of methods and techniques whereby we get a clear sense of genre, and approach the movie with appropriate expectations.

While sitting on the train that day, I felt as if I was living out one of those absurd "mashups" that were popular in the early 2000s, in which mischievous people with a lot of time on their hands took the preview clip of a particular type of movie and overlaid it with the musical score of a completely different type, turning what was once an action flick into a love story, or a horror movie into a slapstick comedy.

But that's what dementia care is like: taking the momentous experience of witnessing a terminal illness and infusing it with cues that we've been trained to associate with a different kind of experience. For those of us who learned about death by watching Leonardo di Caprio exchange a heartfelt farewell with Kate Winslet and then slide below the water in *Titanic*, it's a rude awakening. There's no grand music in the background to stir your spirits. The loved one's clothes and hygiene tend to decline, and the lighting in nursing homes is rarely flattering. Far from deep conversations that resolve lifelong issues, we spend years discussing topics like incontinence and resolving petty quarrels with other residents or with health care providers. The "genre" of dementia, so to speak, may be tragedy; the mode more often resembles satire or surrealism. Above all, death from dementia lasts longer than a movie. While it's happening, it feels like endless weariness, and when it ends it feels too soon.

Modes in Philosophy

Well on into my mother's dementia, her sister came to visit her. Aunt Mary Jane had worked in nursing homes and had seen her fair share of dementia cases. After the visit, she said to me,

"It's clearly an effort for her to come back from her inner place." Her words threw into focus a feeling that had been growing on me for some time: that Mom was spending more and more time in some "hidden place," and that leaving it to interact with the world around her was becoming more and more difficult.

The scholastic philosophers saw "mode" as the means whereby an abstract concept is focused into some concrete form.[5] In this view, the philosopher strives to understand how abstractions, in themselves elusive and difficult to grasp intellectually, show themselves in the world, implicitly assuming that a single abstract concept can be manifested in a multitude of ways. Spinoza went one better, arguing that at the heart of everything lies just one substance – God – that we approach through a variety of modes.[6] All of our ways of understanding and interacting with the world are modes, attempting in their different ways to approach something secret and hidden at the heart of things.

As time went on, I found that both of my parents became more and more mysterious: as if they were both retreating to that "inner place" inside themselves, withdrawing from the everyday world. And we, their children, resorted to different strategies: singing songs, looking through photo albums, telling stories. Each was a mode of approaching something beyond reach.

The Modes in This Book

In the decade or so of caring for our parents, my sisters and I held many, many, many discussions: in person, by phone, on email. And in our discussions, we covered all four of the modes I discuss in this book.

In the early stages, we were heavily in the describing mode. Anxious phone calls took place between us as we gradually realized that Mom and Dad were both acting strangely. What was their condition? Were we dealing with a brain tumor? The effects of sleep apnea? A heart condition? Through seemingly endless consultations with doctors, gerontologists, and specialists of all kinds, we tried to pin down in medical terms what exactly we were dealing with.

As the dementia progressed, these discussions moved into the understanding mode and became increasingly interleaved with consultations about our parents' inner states, sharing insights on how to interpret our mother's increasing aphasia and our father's increasing passivity. In negotiating our parents' transition to assisted living, we learned how to function in the advocating mode, working with doctors, gerontologists, nursing home staff, care directors, specialists, administrators, and hospital staff. And we watched for those moments when the imagining mode took over, such as when our mother's arthritic fingers took to the piano to play familiar songs, or when their cat jumped onto our father's lap, and he stroked her head with a gesture identical to one in old photographs of him as a young boy, with a cat from his childhood. In such times, we relished a sense of familiarity, regularity, and simple friendliness, flourishing in spite of all that was happening to them.

All the time, however, our parents remained mysteries to us, and they defied virtually all of our interpretive efforts.

One afternoon, my father and I were sitting in my sister's house. It had been a difficult few days: our parents had moved out of the family home and were waiting until their apartment in a retirement home became available the following day. My comparatively easy job was to sit with Dad and keep him company while my sisters were getting the apartment ready. Dad had become quite passive and non-communicative, seemingly indifferent to all the change happening around him. Nothing I said seemed to register with him, and I settled for putting on an old episode of *Agatha Christie's Poirot*, with David Suchet. As the familiar story began to unfold, my eyes slowly closed, and I dropped off to sleep in my chair. When I awoke, the episode was well advanced. I looked over and found Dad watching me steadily. "Tired?" he asked quietly. I nodded and smiled, and we both turned back to Poirot.

I've thought many times about that moment: about Dad's quiet, attentive expression and his one-word question. Sometimes I wonder if he was offended at my dropping off to sleep in his presence, and his question showed a resurgence of that terse sarcasm I remember from earlier years. At other times, I wonder if it was the reflex response of a parent, the same reflex that caused him to pull out an empty wallet after we'd taken them out for lunch, on the automatic assumption that he was to pay the bill.

At still other times, I wonder if the answer is simpler: he was watching his son with the love and compassion that formed a large part of his nature.

And sometimes, I wonder if the answer is still simpler: the question meant nothing at all beyond an idle curiosity which was all his brain could muster.

Each of these guesses is a mode, pointing at something I will never know. I can only decide which mode to adopt. Most of the time, I opt for the love and compassion. That was, after all, my father's better self, and my final task as a caregiver is to remember my parents at their best as often as possible.

Notes

Part One: Introduction

1 William Butler Yeats, "The Second Coming," in *The Yeats Reader* (Scribner Poetry, 1997), 80.

Chapter 1: Introducing Dementia Care

1 Mike Barnes, *Be With: Letters to a Caregiver* (Windsor, Ontario: Biblioasis, 2018), 47.
2 Shannon Halloway and Bryan D. James, "A Tsunami of Dementia Could Be on the Way," *Scientific American*, accessed February 5, 2023, https://blogs.scientificamerican.com/observations/a-tsunami-of-dementia-could-be-on-the-way/; Steven R. Sabat, "Dementia in Developing Countries: A Tidal Wave on the Horizon," *The Lancet (British Edition)* 374, no. 9704 (2009): 1805–6, https://doi.org/10.1016/S0140-6736(09)62037-7; World Health Organization, "Dementia," accessed February 5, 2023, www.who.int/news-room/fact-sheets/detail/dementia.
3 Public Health Agency of Canada, "A Dementia Strategy for Canada: Together We Aspire," April 20, 2021, www.canada.ca/en/public-health/services/publications/diseases-conditions/dementia-strategy.html.
4 Canada, "A Dementia Strategy for Canada."
5 Barnes, *Be With*, 15.
6 Barnes, *Be With*, 39.
7 Richard M. Ryan, *Self-Determination Theory: Basic Psychological Needs in Motivation, Development, and Wellness* (New York, New York: The Guilford Press, 2017), 11.
8 Scott O. Lilienfeld et al., *Psychology: From Inquiry to Understanding*, Canadian ed. (Toronto: Pearson Canada, 2011), 3011
9 Lilienfeld et al., *Psychology: From Inquiry to Understanding*, 353.
10 Stephen Sondheim and Hugh Wheeler *A Little Night Music: A New Musical Comedy* (New York: Dodd, Mead, 1973).
11 Samuel Johnson, *A Dictionary of the English Language: In Which the Words Are Deduced from Their Originals*, 1818.

12 "Top 10 George Carlin Quotes – TIME," *Time*, accessed July 27, 2024, https://content.time.com/time/specials/packages/article/
13 Jens-Erik Mai, "Classification in a Social World: Bias and Trust," *Journal of Documentation* 66, no. 5 (2010): 627–42, https://doi.org/10.1108/00220411011066763.

Chapter 2: Introducing Modes

1 *Star Trek*, season 1, episode 10, "The Corbomite Maneuver," written by Jerry Sohl, directed by Joseph Sargenti, aired November 10, 1966, on NBC.
2 Dante, *The Divine Comedy of Dante Alghieri*, trans. John D. Sinclair, vol. 5 (Oxford, 1961), 23.
3 Rebecca Mead, *My Life in Middlemarch* (New York: Broadway Books, 2014).
4 Kyo Maclear, "It Bears Repeating: The Stories We Tell about Dementia – The Globe and Mail," *The Globe and Mail*, 2023, sec. Opinion, www.theglobeandmail.com/opinion/article-it-bears-repeating-the-stories-we-tell-about-dementia/.
5 See Appendix 2 for a further elaboration on modes in music.
6 Northrop Frye, *Words with Power: Being a Second Study of "The Bible and Literature"* (Toronto: Penguin Books, 1990), 4
7 Frye, *Words with Power*, 17
8 Frye, *Words with Power*, 22

Chapter 3: Labelling Dementia

1 Heather Menzies, *Enter Mourning: A Memoir on Death, Dementia, & Coming Home* (Key Porter, 2009), 49.
2 Heather Menzies, "Heather Menzies | Seeker, Writer, Speaker," accessed May 12, 2024, https://heathermenzies.ca/.
3 Ester Carolina Apesoa-Varano, "'I Know Best:' Women Caring for Kin with Dementia," *Social Science & Medicine* 256 (July 1, 2020): 113026, https://doi.org/10.1016/j.socscimed.2020.113026.
4 Menzies, *Enter Mourning*, 51.
5 Thomas Lathrop Stedman, *Stedman's Medical Dictionary [Electronic Resource]*, 28th ed. (Philadelphia: Lippincott Williams & Wilkins, 2006).
6 American Psychiatric Association, *Diagnostic and Statistical Manual of Mental Disorders: DSM-5*, 5th ed. (Arlington, Virginia: American Psychiatric Association, 2013).
7 American Academy of Family Physicians, "Diseases and Conditions," familydoctor.org, 2022, https://familydoctor.org/diseases-and-conditions/.
8 National Library of Medicine, "MedlinePlus – Health Information from the National Library of Medicine," accessed May 12, 2024, https://medlineplus.gov/.
9 National Institute of Neurological Disorders and Stroke, "Dementias," November 6, 2023, www.ninds.nih.gov/health-information/disorders/dementias.
10 Alzheimer's Association, "What Is Alzheimer's?," Alzheimer's Disease and Dementia, 2024, https://alz.org/alzheimers-dementia/what-is-alzheimers.
11 Joseph E. Gaugler et al., "Characteristics of Patients Misdiagnosed with Alzheimer's Disease and Their Medication Use: An Analysis of the NACC-UDS Database," *BMC Geriatrics* 13, no. 1 (December 19, 2013): 137, https://doi.org/10.1186/1471-2318-13-137.

12 American Academy of Family Physicians, "Diseases and Conditions," familydoctor.org, 2022, https://familydoctor.org/diseases-and-conditions/.
13 National Institute of Neurological Disorders and Stroke, "Dementias."
14 National Library of Medicine, "Dementia," Text, Medline Plus, 2021, https://medlineplus.gov/dementia.html.
15 I am grateful to Karen Johnson, director of Outreach Services, McCormick Home, London, Ontario, for making this connection between "dementia" and "dementors" in her presentation at the symposium "Redefining Dementia," that took place in London, Ontario, on April 11, 2015.

Chapter 4: Classifying Dementia

1 National Library of Medicine, "PubMed," PubMed, accessed May 12, 2024, https://pubmed.ncbi.nlm.nih.gov/.
2 National Library of Medicine, "Medical Subject Headings," accessed December 10, 2023.
3 National Cancer Institute, "Biomarker Testing for Cancer Treatment –NCI," October 5, 2017, www.cancer.gov/about-cancer/treatment/types/biomarker-testing-cancer-treatment.
4 Guy M. McKhann et al., "The Diagnosis of Dementia Due to Alzheimer's Disease: Recommendations from the National Institute on Aging-Alzheimer's Association Workgroups on Diagnostic Guidelines for Alzheimer's Disease," *Alzheimer's & Dementia : The Journal of the Alzheimer's Association* 7, no. 3 (May 2011): 263–69, https://doi.org/10.1016/j.jalz.2011.03.005.
5 American Psychiatric Association, *DSM-5*.
6 The NIA-AA Diagnostic Guide specifies five domains rather than six. Like the *DSM-5*, it specifies language, memory, and visuospatial ability but collapse social cognition, complex attention, and executive function into two domains: *personality* and *reasoning*.
7 James M. Ellison, "Medical Conditions That Can Mimic Dementia | BrightFocus Foundation," Alzheimer's Disease Research, 2024, www.brightfocus.org/alzheimers/article/medical-conditions-can-mimic-dementia.
8 Perminder S. Sachdev et al., "Classifying Neurocognitive Disorders: The DSM-5 Approach," *Nature Reviews Neurology* 10, no. 11 (November 2014): 636, https://doi.org/10.1038/nrneurol.2014.181.
9 Ellison, "Medical Conditions That Can Mimic Dementia | BrightFocus Foundation."
10 Sachdev et al., "Classifying Neurocognitive Disorders," 638.
11 Sachdev et al., "Classifying Neurocognitive Disorders," 640.
12 Risk assessment entails the use of big data to determine the likelihood that someone will develop dementia at some future point. Diagnostic standards, however, warn clinicians not to confuse risk factors with pathology. Obesity, for instance, is a risk factor for vascular dementia; however, clinicians are discouraged from using a patient's obesity to infer vascular dementia, but rather to seek evidence that the vascular dementia actually exists, instead of being a mere likelihood. In this form of big data analysis, the distinction between risk factors and pathology becomes blurred.
13 Sachdev et al., "Classifying Neurocognitive Disorders," 637.
14 McKhann et al., "The Diagnosis of Dementia Due to Alzheimer's Disease."

15 Sachdev et al., "Classifying Neurocognitive Disorders."
16 Dan Blazer, "Neurocognitive Disorders in DSM-5," *American Journal of Psychiatry* 170, no. 6 (June 2013): 585–7, https://doi.org/10.1176/appi.ajp.2013.13020179.
17 World Health Organization, "International Classification of Diseases, 11th Edition (ICD-11)," 2019, www.who.int/standards/classifications/classification-of-diseases.
18 McKhann et al., "The Diagnosis of Dementia Due to Alzheimer's Disease."
19 American Psychiatric Association, *DSM-5*.

Chapter 5: Conversation

1 Cathie Borrie, *The Long Hello: Memory, My Mother, and Me* (New York: Simon & Schuster, 2015), 111.
2 Research Institute for Aging, "Understanding Dementia," Schegel-UW Research Institute for Aging, 2022, https://the-ria.ca/wp-content/uploads/2022/06/UnderstandingDementia_Final.pdf, 3.
3 Linda Clare and Pam Shakespeare, "Negotiating the Impact of Forgetting: Dimensions of Resistance in Task-Oriented Conversations between People with Early-Stage Dementia and Their Partners," *Dementia (London, England)* 3, no. 2 (2004): 211–32, https://doi.org/10.1177/1471301204042338.
4 Linda Clare, "Awareness in People with Severe Dementia: Review and Integration," *Aging & Mental Health* 14, no. 1 (2010): 20–32, https://doi.org/10.1080/13607860903421029.
5 Jonathan Crichton and Tina Koch, "Living with Dementia: Curating Self-Identity," *Dementia (London, England)* 6, no. 3 (2007): 365–81, https://doi.org/10.1177/1471301207081570.
6 T. Kitwood, "The Experience of Dementia," *Aging & Mental Health* 1, no. 1 (February 1997): 13–22, https://doi.org/10.1080/13607869757344.
7 Kitwood, "The Experience of Dementia," 16.
8 Murray Alzheimer Research and Education Program, *Managing and Accommodating Responsive Behaviours in Dementia Care* (Waterloo: University of Waterloo, 2005).
9 Steven R. Sabat, *The Experience of Alzheimer's Disease: Life through a Tangled Web* (Oxford: Blackwell, 2001), 51.
10 See for instance Susan Behuniak's study of demeaning metaphors in Susan M. Behuniak, "The Living Dead? The Construction of People with Alzheimer's Disease as Zombies," *Ageing and Society* 31, no. 1 (2011): 70–92, https://doi.org/10.1017/S0144686X10000693.
11 Sabat, *The Experience of Alzheimer's Disease*, 50.
12 Borrie, *The Long Hello*, 91.
13 Jill Manthorpe and Kritika Samsi, "Person-Centered Dementia Care: Current Perspectives," *Clinical Interventions in Aging* 11 (2016): 1733–40, https://doi.org/10.2147/CIA.S104618.
14 Matthew Tieu and Steve Matthews, "The Relational Care Framework: Promoting Continuity or Maintenance of Selfhood in Person-Centered Care," *The Journal of Medicine and Philosophy: A Forum for Bioethics and Philosophy of Medicine* 49, no. 1 (February 1, 2024): 85–101, https://doi.org/10.1093/jmp/jhad044.
15 Tieu and Matthews, "The Relational Care Framework," 85.
16 Tieu and Matthews, "The Relational Care Framework," 92–3.

17 See Nancy Haak, "Maintaining Connections: Understanding Communication from the Perspective of Persons with Dementia," *Alzheimer's Care Quarterly* 3, no. 2 (2002): 116. See also Kristine N Williams, Carissa K Coleman, and Jinxiang Hu, "Determining Evidence for Family Caregiver Communication: Associating Communication Behaviors with Breakdown and Repair," *The Gerontologist*, December 27, 2022, gnac193, https://doi.org/10.1093/geront/gnac193.
18 J.B. Orange, Rosemary B. Lubinski, and D. Jeffery Higginbotham, "Conversational Repair by Individuals With Dementia of the Alzheimer's Type," *Journal of Speech and Hearing Research* 39, no. 4 (1996): 881–95, https://doi.org/10.1044/jshr.3904.881.
19 Alzheimer Society of Canada, "Communicating with People Living with Dementia," Alzheimer Society of Canada, accessed May 23, 2024, https://alzheimer.ca/en/help-support/i-have-friend-or-family-member-who-lives-dementia/communicating-people-living-dementia.
20 J.B. Orange and Angela Colton-Hudson, "Enhancing Communication in Dementia of the Alzheimer's Type," *Topics in Geriatric Rehabilitation* 14, no. 2 (1998): 56–75, https://doi.org/10.1097/00013614-199812000-00007.
21 Marie Y. Savundranayagam and J.B. Orange, "Matched and Mismatched Appraisals of the Effectiveness of Communication Strategies by Family Caregivers of Persons with Alzheimer's Disease," *International Journal of Language & Communication Disorders* 49, no. 1 (2014): 49–59, https://doi.org/10.1111/1460-6984.12043.
22 Orange, Lubinski, and Higginbotham, "Conversational Repair."
23 Catriona Mackenzie, "Embodied Agents, Narrative Selves," *Philosophical Explorations* 17, no. 2 (2014): 154–71, https://doi.org/10.1080/13869795.2014.886363.

Chapter 6: Categories

1 See Tammy Hopper, "Indirect Interventions to Facilitate Communication in Alzheimer's Disease," *Seminars in Speech and Language* 22 (September 2001): 305–16; Nidhi Mahendra, "Direct Interventions for Improving the Performance of Individuals with Alzheimer's Disease," *Seminars in Speech and Language* 22 (September 2001): 291-304"; Orange and Colton-Hudson, "Enhancing Communication"; and Marie Y. Savundranayagam et al., "Communication and Dementia," *Clinical Gerontologist* 31, no. 2 (2007): 47–63.
2 Paul Grice, *Studies in the Way of Words*, First Harvard University Press paperback edition (Cambridge: Harvard University Press, 1991).
3 Elisabeth Ahlsén, "Conversational Implicature and Communication Impairment," in *The Handbook of Clinical Linguistics* (John Wiley & Sons, Ltd, 2008), 32–48, https://doi.org/10.1002/9781444301007.ch2.
4 Ahlsén, "Conversational Implicature and Communication Impairment," 34, 38.
5 Alice Munro, "The Bear Came Over the Mountain," in *Hateship, Friendship, Courtship, Loveship, Marriage: Stories by Alice Munro* (Toronto: McClelland & Stewart, 2001). Kobo.
6 Munro, "The Bear Came Over the Mountain."
7 Borrie, *The Long Hello*, 107.
8 For studies that support the theory of permanent memory loss, see John R. Hodges et al., "Semantic Memory Impairment in Alzheimer's Disease: Failure

of Access or Degraded Knowledge?" *Neuropsychologia* 30, no. 4 (1992): 301–14; Israel Martínez-Nicolás et al., "The Deterioration of Semantic Networks in Alzheimer's Disease," *Exon Publications* (November 21, 2019): 179–91. For the failure of access theory, see Marjorie Nicholas et al., "On the Nature of Naming Errors in Aging and Dementia: A Study of Semantic Relatedness," *Brain and Language* 54, no. 2 (1996): 184–95.

9 Timothy T. Rogers and James L. McClelland, *Semantic Cognition: A Parallel Distributed Processing Approach* (Cambridge, Massachusetts: MIT Press, 2004), 28.

10 Clare Beghtol, "Classification for Information Retrieval and Classification for Knowledge Discovery: Relationships between 'Professional' and 'Naïve' Classifications," *Knowledge Organization* 30, no. 2 (2003).

11 George Eliot, *Daniel Deronda* (Penguin, 1995), 22.

12 Jon-Frederick Landrigan and Daniel Mirman, "The Cost of Switching between Taxonomic and Thematic Semantics," *Memory & Cognition* 46, no. 2 (February 1, 2018): 191–203, https://doi.org/10.3758/s13421-017-0757-5.

13 Alma Au, Agnes S. Chan, and Helen Chiu, "Conceptual Organization in Alzheimer's Dementia," *Journal of Clinical and Experimental Neuropsychology* 25, no. 6 (September 1, 2003): 737–50, https://doi.org/10.1076/jcen.25.6.737.16468.

14 See Eleanor Rosch et al., "Basic Objects in Natural Categories," *Cognitive Psychology* 8, no. 3 (1976): 382–49. See also George Lakoff, *Women, Fire, and Dangerous Things* (University of Chicago Press, 1987).

15 Bénédicte Giffard et al., "The Hyperpriming Phenomenon in Normal Aging: A Consequence of Cognitive Slowing?," *Neuropsychology* 17, no. 4 (2003): 594–601.

16 D. John Done and Tim M. Gale, "Attribute Verification in Dementia of Alzheimer Type: Evidence for the Preservation of Distributed Concept Knowledge," *Cognitive Neuropsychology* 14, no. 4 (June 1997): 547–71, https://doi.org/10.1080/026432997381475.

17 Giffard et al., "The Hyperpriming Phenomenon in Normal Aging," 594.

18 Xuan Le et al., "Longitudinal Detection of Dementia through Lexical and Syntactic Changes in Writing: A Case Study of Three British Novelists," *Literary and Linguistic Computing* 26, no. 4 (December 1, 2011): 435–61, https://doi.org/10.1093/llc/fqr013.

Chapter 7: Facing Out

1 Mike Barnes, *Be With: Letters to a Caregiver* (Windsor, Ontario: Biblioasis, 2018), 107.

2 Hamilton Review of Books, "A Digger After Daylight: In Conversation with Mike Barnes," Hamilton Review of Books, accessed May 29, 2024, http://hamiltonreviewofbooks.com/hrb-interviews-mike-barnes.

3 Barnes, *Be With*, 97.

4 Barnes, *Be With*, 35.

5 Barnes, *Be With*, 32.

6 I should point out, here, that I am using the term "advocacy" solely as intervention on behalf of one person. There is also a growing record of advocacy in the area of dementia care at large that seeks to improve the lot of everyone: advocacy that is carried out not just by family members but by scholars, professional health care providers, and even more important, persons with dementia themselves. If you're interested in that aspect of advocacy, check out Gorazd B. Stokin,

"Advocacy in Dementia," in *Advocacy in Neurology*, ed. Tissa Wijeratne, Sheila Crewther, and David Crewther (Oxford University Press, 2019), 291–302.
7 For a typical example, see Alzheimer Society of Canada, "Long-Term Care Home Checklist" (Alzheimer Society of Ontario, 2016), https://alzheimer.ca/sites/default/files/documents/Long-term-care-home-checklist-Alzheimer-Society_0.pdf.
8 Yasmin Rafiei, "When Private Equity Takes Over a Nursing Home," *The New Yorker*, August 25, 2022, www.newyorker.com/news/dispatch/when-private-equity-takes-over-a-nursing-home.
9 Cameron Graham, Darlene Himick, and Pier-Luc Nappert, "Economic Rents at the End of Life: For-Profit Eldercare and the Myth of Corporate Accountability," in *Handbook of Accounting in Society* (Edward Elgar Publishing, 2024), 415–28.
10 I should point out that abuse, both physical and psychological, can work both ways. While it is not the concern of this book, research is also showing disturbing evidence of resident-to-staff abuse, particularly in dementia wards in understaffed institutions. See for example Elsie Yan et al., "Staff Turnover Intention at Long-Term Care Facilities: Implications of Resident Aggression, Burnout, and Fatigue," *Journal of the American Medical Directors Association* 25, no. 3 (March 1, 2024): 396–402, https://doi.org/10.1016/j.jamda.2023.10.008.
11 World Health Organization, "Abuse of Older People," 2022, www.who.int/news-room/fact-sheets/detail/abuse-of-older-people.
12 Jeffrey E. Hall, Debra L. Karch, and Alex Crosby, "Uniform Definitions and Recommended Core Data Elements for Use in Elder Abuse Surveillance. Version 1.0," US Centers for Disease Control and Prevention, accessed June 8, 2024, https://stacks.cdc.gov/view/cdc/37909.
13 "Wettlaufer," *CTV National News – CTV Television*, June 6, 2018.
14 Alzheimer Society of Canada, "Guidelines for Care: Person-Centred Care of People with Dementia Living in Care Homes," 2011, https://alzheimer.ca/sites/default/files/documents/Guidelines-for-Care_Alzheimer-Society-Canada.pdf.
15 Murray Alzheimer Research and Education Program, *Managing and Accommodating Responsive Behaviours in Dementia Care* (Waterloo: University of Waterloo, 2005).

Chapter 8: Looking In

1 Alan Bennett, *Allelujah!* (London: Faber & Faber, 2018). Part Two. Kobo.
2 Paul Monette, *Borrowed Time: An AIDS Memoir* (Avon, 1988), 30.
3 See Michael Hirst, "Trends in Informal Care in Great Britain during the 1990s," *Health & Social Care in the Community* 9, no. 6 (2001): 348–57, https://doi.org/10.1046/j.0966-0410.2001.00313.x. See also Minna Maria Pöysti et al., "Gender Differences in Dementia Spousal Caregiving," *International Journal of Alzheimer's Disease* 2012 (2012), https://doi.org/10.1155/2012/162960.
4 E.M. Brody, "'Women in the Middle' and Family Help to Older People," *The Gerontologist* 21, no. 5 (October 1, 1981): 471–80, https://doi.org/10.1093/geront/21.5.471.
5 A. Neufeld and M.J. Harrison, "Unfulfilled Expectations and Negative Interactions: Nonsupport in the Relationships of Women Caregivers," *Journal of Advanced Nursing* 41, no. 4 (2003): 323–31, https://doi.org/10.1046/j.1365-2648.2003.02530.x.
6 Menzies, *Enter Mourning*, 40.

7 "How to Honor Caregivers During National Family Caregivers Month," @ NCOAging, accessed June 16, 2024, www.ncoa.org/page/national-family-caregivers-month.
8 "How to Show Appreciation for Your Family Caregiver," CareYaya, accessed June 16, 2024, www.careyaya.org/resources/blog/show-appreciation-for-family-caregivers.
9 Neufeld and Harrison, "Unfulfilled Expectations and Negative Interactions."
10 Borrie, *The Long Hello*, 122.
11 Simon Krutter et al., "Comparing Perspectives of Family Caregivers and Healthcare Professionals Regarding Caregiver Burden in Dementia Care: Results of a Mixed Methods Study in a Rural Setting," *Age and Ageing* 49, no. 2 (February 27, 2020): 199–207, https://doi.org/10.1093/ageing/afz165.
12 Anca M. Miron et al., "Fear of Incompetence in Family Caregivers and Dementia Care Transitions," *The International Journal of Aging and Human Development* 96, no. 4 (June 1, 2023): 447–70, https://doi.org/10.1177/00914150221106075.
13 Borrie, *The Long Hello*, 61.
14 Krutter et al., "Comparing Perspectives of Family Caregivers," 202.
15 George Eliot, *Middlemarch* (Oxford University Press, 1997), 184.
16 H.Y. Ng et al., "The Burden of Filial Piety: A Qualitative Study on Caregiving Motivations amongst Family Caregivers of Patients with Cancer in Singapore," *Psychology & Health* 31, no. 11 (November 1, 2016): 1293–1310, https://doi.org/10.1080/08870446.2016.1204450.
17 Ng et al., "The Burden of Filial Piety."
18 Krutter et al., "Comparing Perspectives of Family."
19 Andrés Losada et al., "Ambivalence and Guilt Feelings: Two Relevant Variables for Understanding Caregivers' Depressive Symptomatology," *Clinical Psychology & Psychotherapy* 25, no. 1 (2018): 59–64, https://doi.org/10.1002/cpp.2116.

Chapter 9: Creative Surges

1 William Butler Yeats, "Sailing to Byzantium" (Scribner 1997), 84.
2 Arthur Laurents, "The Turning Point Movie Script – Page #3," Scripts: The World's Largest Resource for Movie and Play Scripts, 1977, www.scripts.com/script/the_turning_point_22370/3.
3 "Ballerina with Alzheimer's: The Untold Story Of Marta Cinta," November 15, 2020, www.balletherald.com/ballerina-with-alzheimers-marta-cinta/.
4 William W. Beatty et al., "Piano Playing in Alzheimer's Disease: Longitudinal Study of a Single Case," *Neurocase* 5, no. 5 (September 1, 1999): 459–69, https://doi.org/10.1080/13554799908402740.
5 Anne Cowles et al., "Musical Skill in Dementia: A Violinist Presumed to Have Alzheimer's Disease Learns to Play a New Song," *Neurocase* 9, no. 6 (December 1, 2003): 493–503, https://doi.org/10.1076/neur.9.6.493.29378.
6 Oliver Sacks, *Musicophilia: Tales of Music and the Brain* (Knopf, 2007).
7 Kimberlee Speakman, "How Tony Bennett Lived and Sang for Years with Alzheimer's," *People*. Accessed September 6, 2025. https://people.com/how-tony-bennette-lived-sang-for-years-with-alzheimers-desease-7563963.
8 Michael Rossato-Bennett, dir., *Alive Inside: A Story of Music and Memory*, 2014.
9 Anne Davis Basting, Maureen Towey, and Ellie Rose, eds., *The Penelope Project: An Arts-Based Odyssey to Change Elder Care* (Iowa City: University of Iowa Press, 2016), 1.

10 Brigg B. Noyes et al., "Review: The Role of Grief in Dementia Caregiving," *American Journal of Alzheimer's Disease & Other Dementias* 25, no. 1 (February 1, 2010): 9–17, https://doi.org/10.1177/1533317509333902.
11 Hannah Zeilig, John Killick, and Chris Fox, "The Participative Arts for People Living with a Dementia: A Critical Review," *International Journal of Ageing and Later Life* 9, no. 1 (October 9, 2014): 7–34, https://doi.org/10.3384/ijal.1652-8670.14238.
12 Guzmán-Garcia et al., "Dancing as a Psychosocial Intervention in Care Homes: A Systematic Review of the Literature," *Journal of Geriatric Psychiatry* 28, no. 9 (2013): 914–24, https://doi.org/10.1002/gps.3913.
13 Zeilig, Killick, and Fox, "The Participative Arts," 25.
14 Vicky Karkou and Bonnie Meekums, "Dance Movement Therapy for Dementia," *Cochrane Database of Systematic Reviews*, no. 2 (2017), https://doi.org/10.1002/14651858.CD011022.pub2.
15 Sunita R. Deshmukh, John Holmes, and Alastair Cardno, "Art Therapy for People with Dementia," *The Cochrane Database of Systematic Reviews* 9, no. 9 (September 13, 2018): CD011073, https://doi.org/10.1002/14651858.CD011073.pub2.
16 Makiko Abe, Ken-ichi Tabei, and Masayuki Satoh, "The Assessments of Music Therapy for Dementia Based on the Cochrane Review," *Dementia and Geriatric Cognitive Disorders Extra* 12, no. 1 (January 21, 2022): 6–13, https://doi.org/10.1159/000521231.
17 Wen Grace Chen et al., "Music and Brain Circuitry: Strategies for Strengthening Evidence-Based Research for Music-Based Interventions," *Journal of Neuroscience* 42, no. 45 (November 9, 2022): 8498–8507, https://doi.org/10.1523/JNEUROSCI.1135-22.2022.
18 Celia Moreno-Morales et al., "Music Therapy in the Treatment of Dementia: A Systematic Review and Meta-Analysis," *Frontiers in Medicine* 7 (May 19, 2020), https://doi.org/10.3389/fmed.2020.00160.
19 See Jennie L. Dorris et al., "Effects of Music Participation for Mild Cognitive Impairment and Dementia: A Systematic Review and Meta-Analysis," *Journal of the American Geriatrics Society* 69, no. 9 (2021): 2659–67, https://doi.org/10.1111/jgs.17208. See also Sandra Garrido et al., "Music Playlists for People with Dementia: Trialing A Guide for Caregivers," *Journal of Alzheimer's Disease* 77, no. 1 (January 1, 2020): 219–26, https://doi.org/10.3233/JAD-200457 for a discussion of how some playlist programs can have a negative effect if the familiar music triggers traumatic memories.
20 Karyn Stuart-Röhm, Felicity A. Baker, and Imogen Clark, "Training Formal Caregivers in the Use of Live Music Interventions during Personal Care with Persons Living with Dementia: A Systematic Mixed Studies Review," *Aging & Mental Health* 27, no. 10 (February 20, 2023): 1–11, https://doi.org/10.1080/13607863.2023.2180485.
21 Anne Davis Basting, *Forget Memory: Creating Better Lives for People with Dementia* (Baltimore: Johns Hopkins University Press, 2009), 2–3.

Chapter 10: Pleasure

1 Alfred Lord Tennyson, "The Princess," *Tennyson's Poetry*, ed. Robert W. Hill, Jr. (Norton, 1999), 197.

2 William M. Hartmann, *Principles of Musical Acoustics [Electronic Resource]*, 1st ed., Undergraduate Lecture Notes in Physics (New York: Springer New York, 2013), https://doi.org/10.1007/978-1-4614-6786-1.
3 Borrie, *The Long Hello*, 165.
4 Hartmann, *Principles of Musical Acoustics [Electronic Resource]*, 71.
5 Barnes, *Be With*, 60.
6 Munro, "The Bear Came Over the Mountain."
7 Quoted in Craig Zadan, *Sondheim & Co.*, 2nd ed. (New York: Harper & Row, 1986), 231.
8 Siu-Lan Tan, *Psychology of Music: From Sound to Significance*, 2nd ed. (London: Routledge, 2018), 239.
9 Susanne Katherina Knauth Langer, *Philosophy in a New Key: A Study in the Symbolism of Reason, Rite, and Art* (Cambridge: Harvard University Press, 1951), 209.
10 Carroll C. Pratt, *The Meaning of Music: A Study in Psychological Aesthetics*, 1st ed. (New York and: McGraw-Hill Book Company, Inc., 1931).
11 Langer, *Philosophy in a New Key*, 240.
12 Eduard Hanslick, *Eduard Hanslick's On the Musically Beautiful: A New Translation* (New York: Oxford University Press, 2018), Chapter 5. Kobo.
13 Hanslick, *Eduard Hanslick's On the Musically Beautiful*, Chapter 2.
14 Langer, *Philosophy in a New Key*, 228.
15 Leonard B. Meyer, *Emotion and Meaning in Music*. (Chicago: University of Chicago Press, 1956), 35.
16 David Huron, *Sweet Anticipation: Music and the Psychology of Expectation* (The MIT Press, 2006), https://doi.org/10.7551/mitpress/6575.001.0001.
17 Stephen Sondheim, *Finishing the Hat: Collected Lyrics (1954–1981) with Attendant Comments, Principles, Heresies, Grudges, Whines and Anecdotes*, 1st ed. (New York: Knopf, 2010), 71
18 David Leeming, *James Baldwin: A Biography* (Arcade 2015), Chapter 34, Audiobook.
19 Barnes, *Be With*, 103.
20 Menzies, *Enter Mourning*, 91.

Chapter 11: A Skeptical Pause

1 Margaret Laurence, *The Stone Angel* (McClelland & Stewart, 1988), 304–5.
2 George Eliot, *Middlemarch* (Oxford, 1998), 79.
3 Alzheimer Society of Canada, "Learn about the Advisory Group," Alzheimer Society of Canada, accessed July 24, 2024, https://alzheimer.ca/en/take-action/change-minds/advisory-group/learn-about-the-advisory-group.
4 Northrop Frye, *Anatomy of Criticism: Four Essays*, Princeton paperback ed. (Princeton: Princeton University Press, 1971).
5 Joss Whedon, Director's Commentary on "The Body," *Buffy the Vampire Slayer*, Season 5, Episode 94, (20th-Century Fox, 1993).

Chapter 12: An Optimistic Conclusion

1 Haewon Byeon, "Screening Dementia and Predicting High Dementia Risk Groups Using Machine Learning," *World Journal of Psychiatry* 12, no. 2 (February 19, 2022): 204–11, https://doi.org/10.5498/wjp.v12.i2.204.

2 Jiamin Dai, Joan C. Bartlett, and Karyn Moffatt, "Library Services Enriching Community Engagement for Dementia Care: The Tales & Travels Program at a Canadian Public Library as a Case Study," *Journal of Librarianship and Information Science* 55, no. 1 (March 1, 2023): 123–36, https://doi.org/10.1177/0961000621 1065170.
3 Frauke Claes and Paul Enzlin, "Dementia and Sexuality: A Story of Continued Renegotiation," *The Gerontologist* 63, no. 2 (2023): 308–17, https://doi.org/10.1093/geront/gnac127.
4 Daniel J. Levitin, *The World in Six Songs: How the Musical Brain Created Human Nature* (New York: Dutton, 2008), 14.
5 For an example of the wide-ranging research on the neurological aspects of music, see Peter J. Rentfrow et al., *Foundations in Music Psychology: Theory and Research* (Cambridge, Massachusetts: The MIT Press, 2019).
6 Alfred Hitchcock, "The Enjoyment of Fear," *Good Housekeeping* 128, no. 9 (1949): 39–42.
7 Aristotle, "Poetics," in *The Philosophy of Aristotle*, translated by J.L. Creed and A.E. Wardman (Signet, 2011), 471.
8 Roger Scruton, *The Aesthetic Understanding: Essays in the Philosophy of Art and Culture* (Manchester: Carcanet Press, 1983), 87.

Epilogue

1 Gerald Moore, *Am I Too Loud: Memoirs of an Accompanist* (London: Hamish Hamilton, 1962), 202.
2 Moore, *Am I Too Loud*, 46.

Appendix 2: More about Modes

1 John Heil, "Accidents, Modes, Tropes, and Universals," *American Philosophical Quarterly* 51, no. 4 (2014): 338.
2 Plato, *The Republic of Plato*, translated, with notes and an interpretive essay, by Allan Bloom (New York: Basic Books, 1968), 77.
3 Carol J. Williams, "3 Modes and Manipulation: Music, the State, and Emotion," in *Ordering Emotions in Europe, 1100–1800*, vol. 195, Studies in Medieval and Reformation Traditions, 2015, 48–68.
4 F.R. Palmer, *Mood and Modality*, 2nd ed., Cambridge Textbooks in Linguistics (Cambridge: University Press, 2001), 2.
5 Simon Blackburn, *The Oxford Dictionary of Philosophy*, 2nd revised edition (Oxford: University Press, 2008), 236.
6 Benedictus de Spinoza, *Ethics*, Oxford Philosophical Texts (Oxford: Oxford University Press, 2000).

Index

abuse, physical and psychological, 211n10
Advisory Group of People with Lived Experience of Dementia, 162
advocacy: family caregiver, 98–9; term, 210n6
advocating mode, 27–8, 93, 164, 203; caregiver support, 112–13; dementia, 174–7, 179; family conflict, 116–18; Frye, 97; research sources, 190; single caregiver, 113–15; stresses of the caregiver, 115
Agatha Christie's Poirot (television show), 204
aging population, Canada, 100
Ahlsén, Elizabeth, 81–2
AIDS epidemic, 114
Alexa, 86
Alive Inside (film), 133, 135, 136, 138, 139, 147
allegiance, 111

Allelujah! (Bennett), 112
Alzheimer's Association, 42
Alzheimer's disease, 35, 42, 44, 66, 133, 182; cause, 42; death with, 43; dementia type, 85; diagnosis of, 39, 55; NIA-AA guidelines, 50; subtype, 54; term, 36, 42
Alzheimer societies, 28, 101, 118, 134, 171
Alzheimer Society, guidelines for person-centered approach, 109
Alzheimer Society of Canada, 78, 101, 162; checklist, 101–2
ambiguous loss, 136
ambivalence, definition, 125
American Academy of Family Physicians, 41, 43
American Air Force song, 73
American Psychological Association, 189
Am I Too Loud? (Moore), 182
Anatomy of Criticism (Frye), 163
Aricept, term, 36

Aristotle, 178, 200
art(s), 20–3; creative therapy, 142; miracle of, 132–6
artificial intelligence, 169
assessment, term, 36
assisted care, images of, 99–102
assisted living: dementia care, 7; nightmare at the bedside, 103–5; nightmare at the corporate level, 102–3
Asti (formerly Sienna Living), 100
As You Like It (Shakespeare), 45
Ativan, term, 36
Austen, Jane, 152

Bach, 181
Baldwin, James, 152
Bancroft, Anne, 129
Barnes, Mike, 5, 11, 15, 16, 30, 95–7, 146, 153
Basting, Anne Davis, 134, 141, 177
"Bear Came Over the Mountain, The" (Munro), 83, 146
Beethoven, 131, 181
"being-in-the-world," 62
Bennett, Alan, 112
Bennett, Tony, 133
Be With (Barnes), 15, 95, 96
Bible, 19, 20
big data, 169; risk assessment, 207n12
biomarkers, dementia, 49–50, 55
Blake, William, 20
Borrie, Cathie, 15, 16, 30, 65–7, 71, 74, 77, 83, 114, 117, 120, 122, 144, 153, 154
Brahms, organ postlude, 184
Brody, Elaine, 116
Bronte, Charlotte, 44
Buffy the Vampire Slayer (television show), 165
Bute, Jennifer, 67, 161

Calloway, Cab, 134, 148, 149
Canada: aging population, 100; dementia strategy, 7, 8–9, 118; National Dementia Strategy, 7
caregiver(s): advocating mode, 98, 174–7; assistance, 15–18; bond with one being cared for, 160–1; commitments, 100–1; family conflict, 116–18; from the problem to the person, 70–7; images of assisted care, 99–102; inner limits, 123–5; loyalty and allegiance, 111; meaning music, 147–9; memory challenges, 85–6; music as connection, 143–5; music interventions, 139; outer limits of, 120–3; primary problems as, 119–20; responsibility of, 152–5; retirement homes, 126; sanctity, 118–20; single, in advocating mode, 113–15; stresses of, 115; understanding patient, 68–70. *See also* family caregiver(s)
Caregiver Action Network, 118
caregiving: ambivalence, 125; Borrie's experience, 66; memoir of, 11; relationship of music to, 151–2; waking challenges, 105–8
Care Y-AYA Health Alliance, 119
Carlin, George, 14
catharsis, term, 178
cause, dementia, 41–2
Chartwell, 100
ChatGPT, 187
checklist, Alzheimer Society of Canada, 101–2
Christian Gospels, 139
Christie, Agatha, 21, 91, 168
Churchill, Winston, 27
CINAHL database, 190
Cinta, Marta, 129–32, 138, 139

classification of dementia, 164; binary divisions *vs* continuous variables, 58–9; cognitive approaches, 50–2; diagnosis, 53–6; disciplinary roots, 48–52; medical context *vs* social context, 59–60; neurological approaches, 49–50; qualitative *vs* quantitative measurement, 58; vocabulary, 56–8
Cochrane Library, 137
cognition, term, 36
cognition domains, *DSM-5*, 50–2
cognitive approaches, dementia, 50–2
cognitive economy, 13
cognitive impairment, 33
cognitive psychology, simple in, 88–9
coherence, 13, 160; concept of, 167; need for, 13–15, 167–8
collaboration, understanding patient, 68–70
commitment to positive change, 179
communication, loss of, and caring process, 92
communication research: repairing what's broken, 77–9. *See also* conversation
communication researchers, simple language and syntax, 80–1
community-based dementia care, 170
complex attention, cognition domain, 51
conceptual/dialectic mode, Frye's, 66–7
connection, music, 144
conspiracy theory, 194
conversation: communication research, 77–9; from the outer world to the inner world, 67–70; from the problem to the person, 70–7; implicatures, 81–4; maxims of, 81–2; repairing what's broken, 77–9
conversational repair, 77–8
COVID pandemic, 6, 28, 103; caregiver initiatives, 118–19; elder care, 175–6
creative arts, 143
"creative care" approach, 134
creativity: artistry of music and dance, 129–32; evidence, 136–40; miracle of art, 132–6; modes, 29
cultural landscape, dementia, 22
curation, term, 69–70
curiosity sensations, 179

daily life: dementia in terms of, 60; real world, 37–8
dance, creative therapy, 142
Dante, 20, 21, 23, 178
DeBaggio, Thomas, 161
Deci, Edward, 12
declarative memory, 84–5
definition, dementia, 40–1
dementia: advocating mode, 174–7; art therapy, 138; cause, 42; challenge of caring for loved one, 24; cognitive psychology, 88–9; conversational repair, 77–8; definition, 40–1, 52, 54, 60; descriptive mode, 168–71; diagnosis of, 43–4; framing of, 70–7; help for, 15–18; imaginative mode, 177–9; music therapy, 135, 138, 139, 140; need for meaning, 153; normal *vs* abnormal, 42–4; real-life phenomenon, 21–2; single caregiver, 113–15; stages of, 182; symptom *vs* cause, 41–2; understanding mode, 171–4; vocabulary, 44–6

dementia care: "advocacy,"
    210n6; advocating mode, 27–8;
    community-based, 170; demands
    on caregiver, 162; descriptive
    mode, 25–6; experiences, 163;
    families, 17; families to the
    rescue, 6–8; family conflict,
    116–18; family members, 165–6;
    imaginative mode, 28–9; life
    after, 165–6; modes, 30–1; need
    for information, 8–12; normality
    in, 184–5; participatory arts,
    137, 140–1; personal, 5–6;
    phenomenon of, 22; progression
    of seasons, 164; "retreat under
    fire," 111; role of stress in, 136;
    sharing moments of connection,
    178–9; understanding mode, 26–7
dementia cases: coherence, 14–15;
    long-standing "issues," 161
dementia diagnosis: binary divisions
    vs cognitive variables, 58–9;
    medical context *vs* social context,
    59–60; process, 61–2
dementia research, 85; advice,
    192–4; advocating mode, 190;
    being active and not passive,
    187–8; descriptive mode, 189;
    family caregiver, 187–94; filtering
    search results, 190–2; knowledge
    organization principles, 5–6;
    limitations of, 160–3; sources of
    research, 188–90; studies, 16–17;
    understanding mode, 189
dementia strategy, Canada, 7, 8–9,
    118
dementors, Harry Potter books, 44
descriptive/describing mode, 25–6,
    33, 67, 164, 202–3; dementia,
    46–7, 168–71, 178–9; diagnosis of
    dementia, 43–4, 60–2; research

sources, 189; what is happening,
    38–40
Devil Wears Prada, The (film), 68
Dewey's Decimal Classification, 87
diagnosis, dementia, 53–6
*Diagnostic and Statistical Manual
    (DSM)*, defining dementia, 41
*Diagnostic and Statistical Manual
    fifth edition (DSM-5)*: domains
    of cognition, 50–2; major
    neurocognitive disorders, 57,
    59, 60; mild neurocognitive
    disorders, 59, 60; neurocognitive
    disorder, 52; process of diagnosis,
    53; qualitative *vs* quantitative
    measurement, 58; sub-types of
    dementia, 54–5
di Caprio, Leonardo, 201
disabling, term, 43
disorientation, dementia, 41
Divine Comedy (Dante), 21
driving safety, 10

1812 Overture (Tchaikovsky), 148
elder abuse, categories, 104
elder-care residences, Canada, 107
Eliot, George, 21, 29, 123, 159
emotional impairment, dementia, 41
Enter Mourning (Menzies), 15,
    35, 187
Enterprise (starship), 21, 24
episodic memory, 84
Eroica symphony, 131
"errorless training," 80
etiology, dementia, 41–2
executive function, cognition
    domain, 51–2
Extendicare, 100

Facebook, 118
Fake News, 193

family caregiver(s): advocacy,
  98–9; advocating mode,
  175–7; appreciation for, 119;
  dementia, 6–8, 162; life after
  care, 165–6; listening, 182;
  researching dementia as, 187–94;
  understanding patient, 68–9, 79.
  See also caregiver(s)
family conflict, dementia care, 116–18
family members, dementia and, 161–2
Four Seasons (Vivaldi), 148
fronto-temporal, term, 36
frontotemporal dementia, cause, 42
Frye, Northrop, 19–20, 23, 25, 26, 29,
  30, 66, 131, 163

general culture impatience,
  dementia care, 22
"genre," dementia, 201
geriatrician, term, 36
geriatric sexuality, 10
Good Housekeeping (magazine), 178
Google Scholar, 189, 192
grammar, modes in, 198–9
Great Code, The (Frye), 19
Grice, Paul, 81, 82
Gypsy (musical), 151–2

Hamlet (Shakespeare), 6, 22
Hanslick, Eduard, 150
Hard Times (Dickens), Blackpool in,
  13, 15
harmonics: concept of, 145–6; music,
  145–7
Harry Potter books, dementors in, 44
health care systems, dementia on
  rise, 6–7
Heidegger, Martin, 62
helplessness, language and, 80
hepatic encephalopathy (HE), 33
Hitchcock, Alfred, 178

hospice, term, 36
human rights, 108
Huntington's disease, form of
  dementia, 55
"hyperpriming," 90

Ideal Husband, An (Wilde), 93
imaginative literature, 20–3
imaginative/imagining mode, 28–9,
  127, 155, 164, 203; caregiver and,
  179; creativity of caregiver, 141;
  dementia, 177–9
implicatures: conversation, 81–4;
  term, 82
implicit memory, 84
incompetence, sense of, pressure
  point, 121–2
information, precision *vs* simplicity,
  89–91
Instagram, 118
International Classification of
  Diseases (ICD), 60, 62
iPod playlist programs, 138, 139
ischemic, term, 36
isolation, pressure point, 122
isomorphism, term, 148

Jane Eyre (Bronte), 44, 46
Jane Fonda Workout Book, The, 19
Jenkins, Florence Forest, 143
Johnson, Samuel, 14
Journal of Medicine and Philosophy, 75
Joyce, James, 23

Kant, Immanuel, 135
King, Martin Luther, Jr., 27
King Lear (Shakespeare), 124
Kitwood, Thomas, 70, 72
knowledge organization, 20, 86;
  dementia research, 5–6, 23; naïve
  classification, 86–8

Langer, Susanne, 148, 150
language: cognition domain, 50; precision *vs* simplicity, 89–91
Laurence, Margaret, 157
Law and Order (television show), 22
learning and memory, cognition domain, 50
Levitin, Daniel, 177
Lewy body: cause, 42; term, 36
Lewy body disease, diagnosis of, 55; subtype, 54
Lightfoot, Gordon, 131
LinkedIn, 118
listening, understanding mode, 91, 173
literary studies, modes in, 200–1
Little Night Music, A (musical), 13–14
"living death," zombie narratives of, 73
living wills, 10
Long Hello, The (Borrie), 15, 65, 66

Macfie Sobol, Julie, 161
McGowin, Diana Freel, 161
Mackenzie, Catriona, 79
Maclear, Kyo, 22
major neurocognitive disorder, 54; DSM-5 diagnosis of, 57; term, 45–6
Matthews, Steve, 75, 76
Maurois, Andre, 172
Mead, Rebecca, 21
meaning, need for, 153
Meaning of Music, The (Pratt), 149
medical context, dementia diagnosis, 59–60
Medline Plus, 188, 189
memory, lost or mislaid, 84–6
mental disorder, National Library of Medicine, 48–9
mental illness, Barnes on, 95–7

mental impairment, dementia, 41
Menzies, Heather, 15, 16, 30, 35–6, 39, 43, 46, 61, 114, 117, 153, 154, 187
Merchant of Venice, The (Shakespeare), 90
metaphor, limitations of, 163–4
Middlemarch (Eliot), 21, 123, 159
minor neurocognitive disorder, 54
miracle cure, 193; approach, 177
Mitchell, Joni, 131
MOCA test, term, 36
"mode": concept, 23–4; definition, 196; term, 195–6, 198
modes: advocating, 27–8, 203; describing, 25–6, 202–3; description of, 23–31; Frye's theory of, 23; grammar, 198–9; imagining, 28–9, 203; literary studies, 200–1; music, 197–8; philosophy, 201–2; understanding, 26–7, 203
"moments of being," Woolf, 154
Monette, Paul, 114
money management, 10
Montreal Cognitive Assessment (MoCA), 53
Moore, Gerald, 182
"muddle," coherence, 13–15
Munro, Alice, 83, 146
Murdoch, Iris, 91
music: caregiver's responsibility, 152–5; creative therapies, 142–3; harmonics, 145–7; making, 143–5; meaning of, 147–9; modes in, 197–8; principles of, 133; pulse of, 149–51; qualities, 144; relationship to caregiving, 151–2; "unconsummated symbol," 149
Música para Despartar, music program, 130
Musicophilia (Sacks), 133

music therapy, 135, 140; dementia,
  135, 138, 143
myth, 163

naïve classifications, 86–8
National Dementia Strategy,
  Canada, 7
National Family Caregivers Month,
  November, 118
National Institute of Neurological
  Disorders and Stroke, 41, 43
National Library of Medicine (NLM),
  43, 189; *Medical Subject Headings*
  (MeSH), 48–9; MEDLINE, 48;
  Medline Plus, 41, 188, 189; mental
  disorder (F03), 48; nervous system
  disease (C10), 48
NCOA. *See* US National Council on
  Aging
need for information, dementia care,
  8–12
nervous system disease, National
  Library of Medicine, 48–9
neurocognitive disorder,
  definition, 52
neurological approach, dementia,
  49–50
neuropsychology, descriptive
  mode, 56
New Yorker, The (magazine), 102
NIA-AA, qualitative *vs* quantitative
  measurement, 58
NIA-AA guidelines, 57, 58;
  Alzheimer's disease, 50
"normal aging," 168
normality, dementia care, 184–5
*Norton Anthology of English
  Literature*, 20

objective truth, descriptive mode,
  25–6

Odyssey (Homer), 200
Order of Canada, Menzies, 35
organist, learning from an, 181–5
overtones, music, 145
Oxford English Dictionary (OED),
  44–5, 70, 195

PAIS (Public Affairs Information
  Service) Index, 190
Parkinson's disease, form of
  dementia, 55
participatory arts: dementia, 143;
  dementia care, 137, 140–1
perceptual-motor function, cognition
  domain, 51
personal care, policy manuals,
  108–11
person-centered care, 75; dementia,
  72; miracle of art, 132–6
"personhood," 75, 76
philosophy, modes in, 201–2
physical abuse, 211n10
PIECES Framework, 110
pitch, music, 144
Plato's *Republic*, 196
Poirot, Hercule, Christie's, 21, 22, 168
policy manuals, personal care level,
  108–11
Porter, Cole, 151
Pratt, Caroll, 149
precision, simplicity *vs*, 89–91
primary progressive aphasia, 182;
  term, 36
priming effects, 90
Princess, The (Tennyson), 142
privacy, 10
procedural memory, 84, 85
PSW, term, 36
psychological abuse, 211n10
psychology: descriptive mode, 56;
  "theory theory," 86–7

PsycInfo database, 189
PubMed, research database, 188, 189

real world, 37–8; dementia diagnosis, 59–60; descriptive mode, 25–6, 38–40
reference librarians, 11
Republic (Plato), 196
research: dementia, 16–18. *See also* dementia research
respite care, 122
responsive behavior, pressure point, 121
retention, signs of, 71
retirement homes, rhetoric of, 126
retirement living, images of assisted care, 99–102
Revera, 100
"rhetoric" mode, 97
risk assessment, 207n12
Romeo and Juliet (Shakespeare), 131
Room with a View, A (Forster), 13
Rosch, Eleanor, 88
Rossato-Bennett, Michael, 133
Russell, Bertrand, 67
Russell, Yvonne, 139–40
Ryan, Richard, 12

Sabat, Steven, 72–4
Sacks, Oliver, 133, 135
"Sailing to Byzantium" (Yeats), 127
St. Mark's Anglican Church, 183
sanctity, dementia care, 118–20
satisfaction: aesthetic experience, 150; qualities of, 150; term, 149
"Scarborough Fair/Canticle" (Simon and Garfunkel), 197
scientific method, empirical research, 170
Scruton, Roger, 179
search engines, 86

"second childhood," 89
Second World War, 27
self-determination theory, sense of competence, 12–13
"selfhood," 76, 88; preserving, 92
semantic memory, 84
senile dementia, term, 44–5
sense of competence, need for, 12–13
sexuality, understanding mode, 173
Shakespeare, William, 45, 63, 90, 116, 131
Shakespeare's Henry V, 27
Share the Care, 118
Shaw, Bernard, 105
signs of neglect, dementia, 172
Simon and Garfunkel's "Scarborough Fair/Canticle," 197
simple, describing, 88–9
simple language, 80–1
simple words, precision *vs* simplicity, 89–91
simplicity, precision *vs*, 89–91
Siri, 86
skepticism, 159, 170, 193
Sobol, Ken, 161
social cognition, cognition domain, 51
social context, dementia diagnosis, 59–60
"Social Sharables," 118
Socrates, 26, 196
Sondheim, Stephen, 148, 151
speech rate, 80
Spinoza, Baruch, 202
stability, music, 144
Star Trek (television show), 19
Star Wars (film), theme of, 197
Stedman's Medical Dictionary, dementia, 41
Stone Angel, The (Laurence), 157
Streep, Meryl, 68
Suchet, David, 204

sundowning, term, 36
Swan Lake (Tchaikovsky), 130, 131
symptom, dementia, 41–2

Tchaikovsky, 148
Tennyson, 155; *The Princess*, 142
"theory theory," 86–7
"thinking outside the box," 194
Tieu, Matthew, 75, 76
Titanic (film), 201
Titus Andronicus (Shakespeare), 19
Turning Point, The (movie), 129
Twitter, 118

Ulysses (Joyce), 23
understanding mode, 26–7, 63, 66, 91–2, 164, 203; dementia, 171–4, 179; research sources, 189
United Church, 183
University of Toronto, 196
US Centers for Disease Control and Prevention, 104
US National Council on Aging, 118
US National Library of Medicine, 188

vascular, term, 36
vascular dementia, 207n12; subtype, 54
Vivaldi, 148
vocabulary: classification and, 56–8; dementia, 44–6
volume, music, 144

Western culture, 10
Wettlaufer, Elizabeth, 104
Whedon, Joss, 165
Wikipedia, 86
Wilde, Oscar, 93, 105, 193
Williams, Carol, 198
Williams, Vaughan, 148
Winslet, Kate, 201
Winter's Tale, The (Shakespeare), 63
Woolf, Virginia, 154
Words with Power (Frye), 25, 66
Wordsworth, William, 154
World Health Organization, 6, 104

Yeats, William Butler, 3, 127